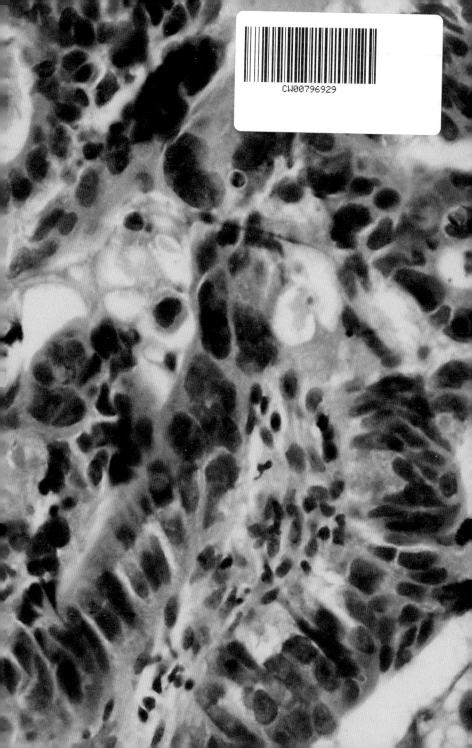

It's Inside

It's Inside

Katharine Meynell & Alistair Skinner

MARION BOYARS PUBLISHERS
LONDON • NEW YORK

Published in Great Britain and the United States in 2005 by
MARION BOYARS PUBLISHERS LTD
24 Lacy Road, London, SW15 1NL

www.marionboyars.co.uk

Distributed in Australia and New Zealand by Peribo Pty Ltd, 58 Beaumont Road,
Kuring-gai, NSW 2080

Printed in 2005
10 9 8 7 6 5 4 3 2 1

A CIP catalogue record for this book is available from the British Library.
A CIP catalog record for this book is available at the Library of Congress.

ISBN 0-7145-3108-1

This book was published with the assistance of Middlesex University.
With thanks to The Wellcome Trust for their invaluable support.

Printed in China

For our children, Paul and Hannah
who grew up through this time and whose joie de vivre has kept life
sweet in so many ways.

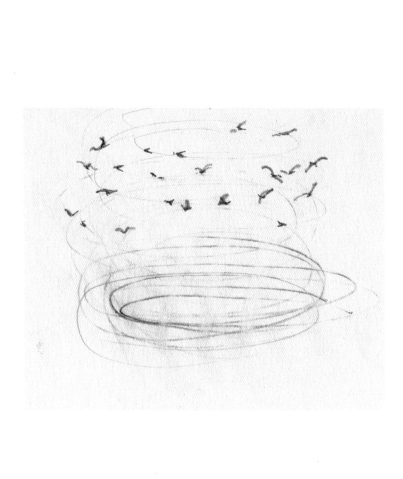

It's Inside – a work towards articulating an experience of disease

So much of Alistair's illness was not discernible. The beginning of the process of articulating an experience of disease was a partial response to the unseen 'cast' that the diagnosis had placed on him. I suppose that this changed in the last three months of his life, where many signs were obvious. Not only did the disease then produce externally observable physical changes, Alistair also began to find ways of describing his sense of this.

We understood that this project would also imply questions of a wider context, necessarily touching on biomedical, aesthetic, ethical and emotional concerns. Many of these also changed our perceptions of the world, taking on a new sharpness. Where the debates over 'cost effectiveness' of drugs personally available on the NHS would be seen in a global landscape of profit and availability. Against this complex background the images we were looking for needed to be sensate and questioning. Disciplinary conventions of representation tend to fail to address issues outside of their boundaries; but although medical imaging processes serve different functions from images that require a less confined interpretation, these were crucial to forming our understanding of the illness. And beyond that, all the different ways of imaging disease can be understood as also containing structures of power in both the looking and the looked at.

We are following a conceptual tradition of art practice in which personal histories overlap the wider realm of social and aesthetic ideas, through (our particular) practice of everyday life. We use extracts from sketchbooks, videos, diaries and other things we collected in an attempt to make some kind of meaning.

A recoding would need to index hybridity as a site shot through and traced with the untranslatable which serves as its supplement and prop. The upshot of this is to dramatise the incomplete, unfixed nature of the category. We begin to see hybridity not so much as a self-standing, fixed term but as an interdependent one — changing and rechanging as it interacts with the aura of the untranslatable, with the remains and leftovers of the translation exercise. These need to be accounted for and acknowledged at every turn, for, to use Adorno's words, like blood stains in a fairytale, they cannot be rubbed off.

Bowel polyps are common; not all are cancerous. They are fleshy out growths from the mucosa of the bowel which is highly glandular tissue. The polyps (and cancers) have a lot of vessels, are easily damaged and bleed.

Liver function impairment produces flu-like symptoms and night sweats. The tumour itself produces cytokines and other factors that could cause these symptoms.

Liver enlargement is due to metastases (secondary tumour deposits from bowel cancer) and secondary inflammatory reaction.

Not sure about voice change. Possibly due to generalised muscle weakness.

I want to write down all the perceptible (to me) traces of illness before I forget them. I would like to know what they each mean, as a parallel text, as a pathology.

Remembering symptoms not mentioned later in the diary

Bleeding from the bowel was an early symptom (it happened when we were still living at Boleyn Road, so that was at least six years ago). Alistair enjoyed reading the paper on the toilet, we assumed the blood was due to the effort of this.

For about two years before diagnosis (March 2001), he had a dragging tiredness accompanied by sporadic 'flu' symptoms and night sweats, which got progressively heavier, leaving what he described as a 'scene of the crime' body outline in our bed. His urine was very dark, he insisted it was 'normal', but it was not like mine. Then his liver grew very large extending well below his rib cage and that was about the time he eventually got a diagnosis. During treatment these symptoms came and went, as the different chemotherapy drugs helped – and then no longer helped.

Alistair felt his voice had changed & he would no longer sing to me. He wouldn't let me listen to him trying, so I don't know in what way it had altered, certainly the talking voice got lower and weaker at times.

Not enough liver tissue to detoxify the alcohol.

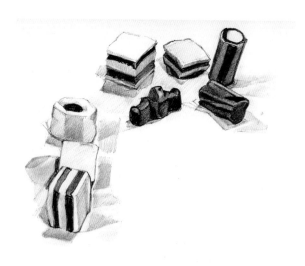

Chemotherapy had worked for a year, or at least the combination of drugs, and holidays, and good times, and work things – all appeared to make a difference to his health in about equal measure. But by June 2002 it was apparent that it was not going to be possible to go on delaying the progression of disease. He had started to loose weight and did not want to drink more than a 'sip for the taste' of alcohol. Alistair, who liked to get drunk as a skunk on Friday night.

We are lucky to be surrounded by doctors (in addition to the ones at the hospital): Paul, Alistair's brother; Eric, Alistair's friend from way back student days; and boho Astrid and Henryk who we met in our 'local', watching the cup final.

We looked into various options for clinical trials, and considered one at the Marsden, but by then Alistair was not in good enough health to be eligible. Henryk (who works in cancer research) asked around internationally about any promising trials, but there was nothing really significant, so at least we knew Alistair had not missed out on anything he could have benefited from.

Concentration fluctuated, in 2001 (with the first bout of chemo) time spent on the ward allowed Alistair space to read voraciously at each treatment, the next year he found he could not read a whole book, we have piles of bought but unread ones. In hospital in July, he gradually found it too hard to read the paper himself, he liked me to read it to him. Then when he got home he watched a lot of sport, had the radio and TV on for the cricket (simultaneously, TV for pictures and radio for the commentary he preferred) as a kind of backdrop. Then he stopped watching anything and no longer wanted the sound context although he never minded if I wanted it. The last two months we retreated into the house, going out only for things we really thought special. Then in the last two weeks we retreated into the bedroom, and then we just stayed in bed.

Immunological response impaired; capacity to fight infection much reduced.

Bacteria:
Gram positive: many are harmless and live usually non-pathogenically, but can cause serious infection (staph / streptococcus) – skin, throat.
Gram negative: (e-coli) – bowel.

There may have been small cesses on the liver. It is also possible that some of the metastases necrosed.

Probably fibrosis, the body's walling off of foreign material. (Or skin metastasis?)

ASCITIS = *abnormal accumulation of liquid from the blood in the peritoneal cavity. The causes of malignant ascites could be as follows:*
'central' form: *the tumour/metastasis invades the liver tissue resulting in compression of the lymphatic and/or portal venous system (big vein very close to and derived from the liver); therefore there is an elevated hydrostatic pressure combined with decreased oncotic pressure; the latter is more the result of limited protein intake and the catabolic state associated with cancer rather than defective hepatic protein synthesis (mainly albumin).*

'peripheral' form: *deposits of tumour cells are found on the surface of the parietal and visceral peritoneum; the ascitis is largely the result of mechanical interference with venous and/or lymphatic drainage, but in this instance the blockage is rather at the level of the peritoneal space rather than the liver parenchyma. Experimentally, reduced efflux of peritoneal fluid precedes increased fluid influx. There are data suggesting that vasoactive substances released from the peritoneal tumour implants and non-malignant monocytes or macrophages increase capillary permeability and thereby contribute to ascitis formation even in the absence of lymphatic obstruction.*

'mixed' form: *in which tumour is present both in the liver and on the peritoneal surface.*
chylous malignant ascitis: *where the tumour of the retroperitoneal space causes obstruction of lymphatic flow through the lymph nodes and/or pancreas. Leakage of the lymphatic channels as a result of direct tumour invasion may also be operative in this form of malignant ascitis.*

By May 2002 Alistair was utterly exhausted, with little energy for anything except the things he very much wanted which curiously included going to work (teaching at UEL two days a week) and sleeping as much as possible.

He got serious sepsis twice, in June and again in July. The first time the Hickman line was taken out because of fears that the infection might have colonised the plastic (although nurse Danny finally unblocked the spare lumen). Then without enough time to recover properly, he got very sick again a few weeks later. Why did this happen after the line has been removed? I believe the culture was both gram positive and gram negative, so because of that, was it likely that there were lingering bacteria?

There was also some infection coming from the liver itself. This was a frightening image: was his liver was rotting inside him?

Antibiotics apparently cleared it up.

When the Hickman line came out it left 2 painless, small (gristly?) lumps on Alistair's ribs, away from the exit site, we never knew why, it bothered him, he felt marked or damaged by them.

Then ascitis, big swollen belly. We were told how this happened, I think it was something to do with an imbalance of amino acids, but what, why and how, I have forgotten or never quite grasped. The result was a seemingly ever expanding capsule of liquid. It became huge and unbearable. He went into Barts and had it drained off – eight and a half litres the first time. It was a slightly iridescent greeny yellow. I sniffed it, but it didn't smell much of anything. I would have investigated it more but the nurse present definitely considered this inappropriate behaviour and I backed off. The liquid itself is protein (amino acids) but they called it 'dead' protein in that the body could not use it. Presumably it also took precious, usable protein out of use. He was told that this now would be a constant feature of his life. Without particular vanity (he was justifiably always so physically confident) this was very difficult. He did not find his body's vulnerability easy.

Almost certainly nerve compression pain caused by tumour deposits impinging on the nerve going to the leg.

Raising the knee takes the nerve off the stretch and reduces the pain.

Alistair experiences a lot of very severe pain in his gut and down his leg. The hospital thinks it is constipation. That may be partly so, but it carries on, particularly down his right thigh. When we get home he finds that changing position sometimes helps, and he wants to keep the leg warm, getting into the bath when he can, or wrapping it up in extra blankets. He lies with his knee raised and rubs his thigh with his hands. Sometimes he howls. Astrid thinks it is referred neuropathic pain. Amitriptyline sorts this out, it seems like a miracle and we are able to get on with going to exhibitions and the theatre again, albeit with Alistair in a wheelchair.

Morphine enables visualisation and sound equivalents.

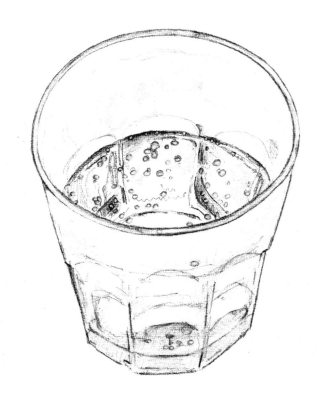

[the] friendship (.18).

Trying to bear witness to a unique friendship without giving in to some narcissistic "we" or "me," being willing to return to the troublesome aspects of the past without wanting to claim the "last word" on it (98), Derrida lays out not so much a middle ground as a series of aporias.

Endoscopy: direct visual examination of the interior of the body by optical viewing instrument. Endoscopes are flexible, usually containing several channels equipped with fibre optics for illumination and viewing. Other channels allow suction, inflation and the means of taking biopsies.

Presumably chest x-ray looking for metastases.

CT delineates lungs, liver retroperitoneum (area outside the lining of abdomen wall). It distinguishes between tissues of different densities.

DIARY etc:

Note book, date unknown, before illness known (Alistair writing)
Build a surface
Frozen moment – still, full focus
Active movement – blur change
Scale
Build an image, element of time in – seeing / making
Inside pushing out – from behind the surface
Out front pushing back into the surface
Alone – image of fragments of isolated parts
Together – touch exploration – enjoyment – love

13th March 2001
Royal Court 3 tickets. Alistair shows Eric blood in toilet.

22nd
Endoscopy. Mr Dorudi, London Hospital 1 pm.
Liver? Inflammatory bowel? Lymphoma? Liver cancer? – biopsy.

26th
10.30 X-ray 1st floor, Alexandra wing.

28th
CT scan 2 p.m.

28th
Mr Dorudi

We walked to the hospital through Haggerston Park. When we finally found the correct clinic (through the labyrinthine architecture) we were ushered into an office, skipping a very, very long queue; Sina Dorudi had his specialist nurse there, who Alistair had met last week.

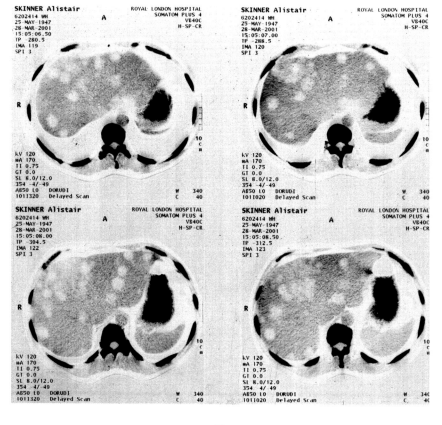

I remember Alistair saying he wanted to see Paul through university and Sina gently telling him that would not happen. Alistair left with a drawing of a colon and metastasised liver, that Sina had done on the back a scrap of perforated computer paper.

Outside, Whitechapel seemed so bright, shimmering. We walked towards the city. Alistair considered going into Covent Garden to the optician, but then decided to go into the Whitechapel Gallery. I have no idea what exhibition was on; I just remember shuffling round in a daze.

Back at home, he crouched on the mezzanine, inconsolably screaming with hot tears. This is the only time I saw him rage about being ill.

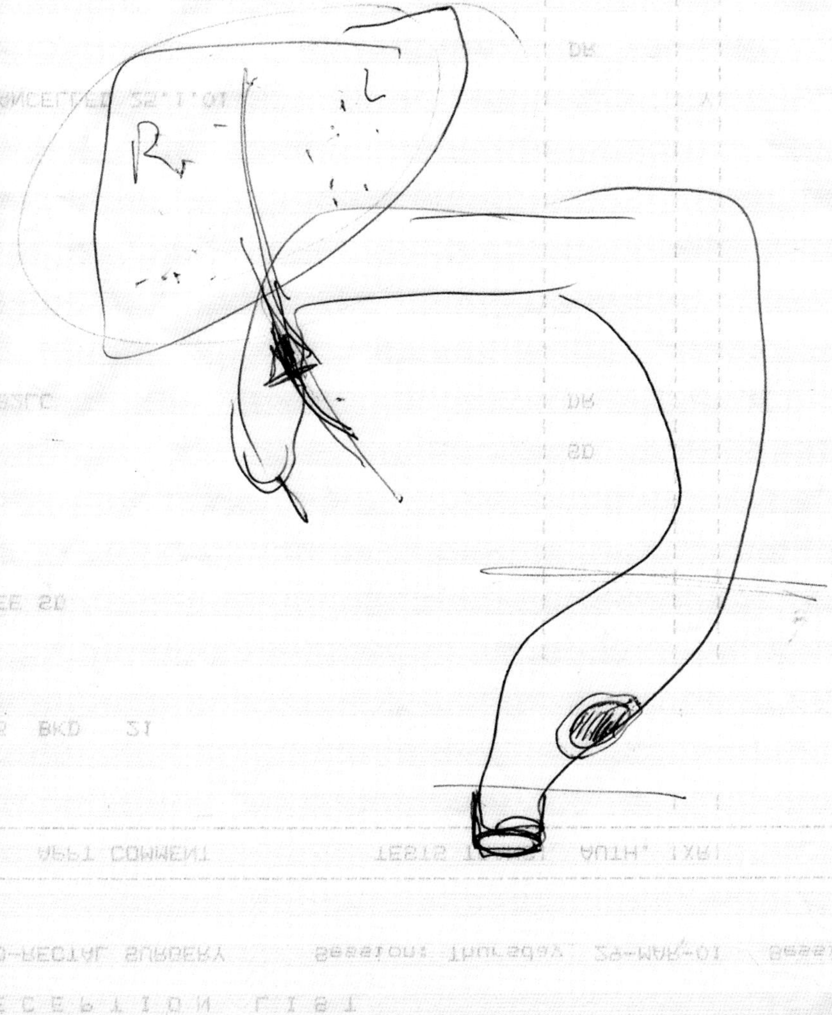

O-RECTAL SURGERY   Session: Thursday 29-MAR-01   Session ID

APPT COMMENT   TESTS T...   AUTH, 1XR!   C

S BKD   21

EE SD

SD

DR   83LC

ANCELLED 25.1.01

DR

DR

SD   4)

PP

APPT	COMMENT	TESTS	TRANS	AUTH.	XR	CLE
BKD	21					
☰ SD						
				SD		
2LC				DR		
ICELLED 25.1.01					Y	
				DR		
				DR		
				SD		
				RP		

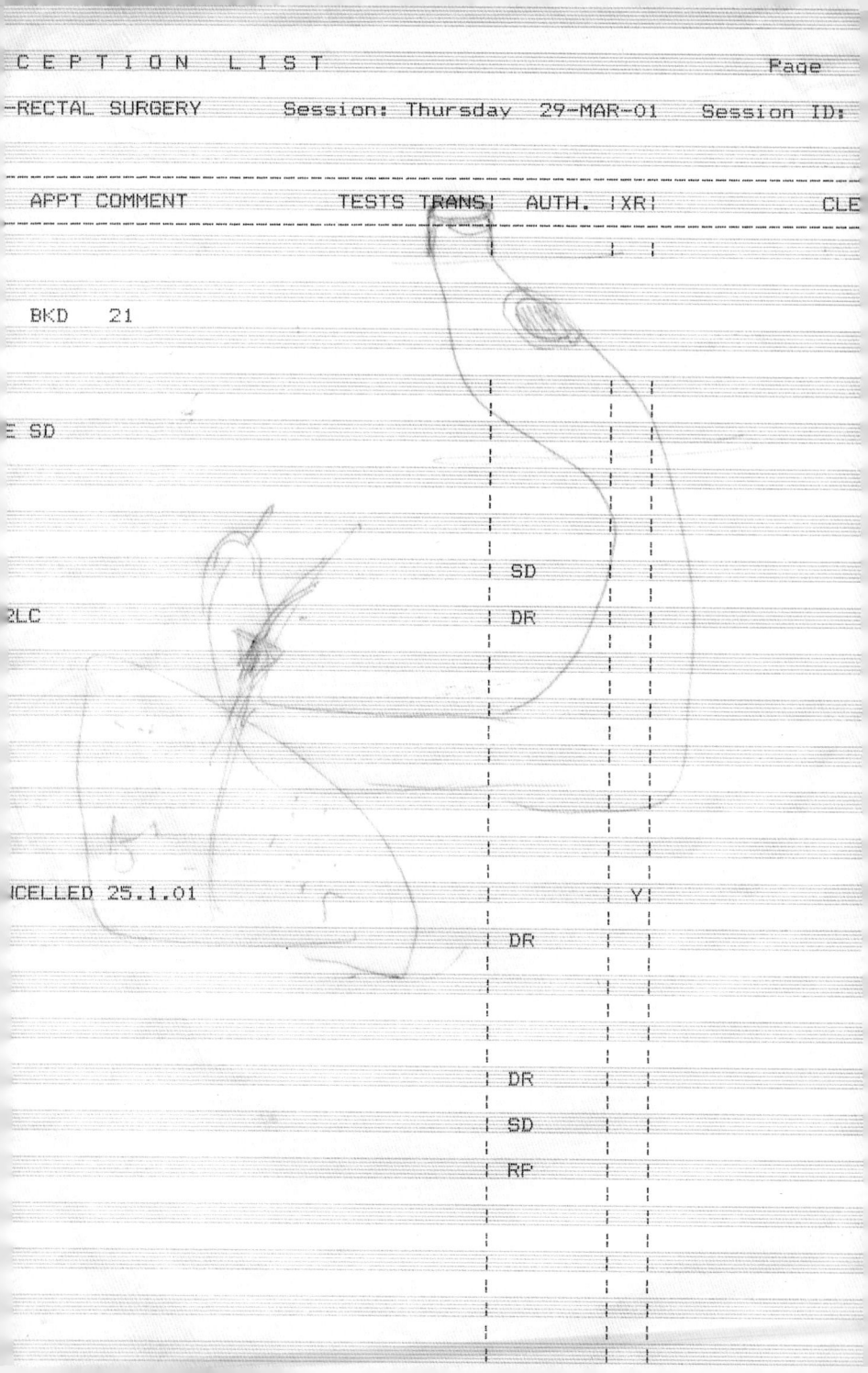

BMJ 2000;321:1278-1281 (18 November)
Clinical review

ABC of colorectal cancer Treatment of advanced disease

Annie Young, Daniel Rea.

Advanced colorectal cancer can be defined as colorectal cancer that at presentation or recurrence is either metastatic or so locally advanced that surgical resection is unlikely to be carried out with curative intent. Despite most patients undergoing potentially curative surgery and the availability of adjuvant chemotherapy, about 50% of patients presenting with colorectal adenocarcinoma die from subsequent metastatic disease. The five year survival rate for advanced colorectal cancer is lower than 5%. In the past few years several therapeutic advancesunderpinned by multiprofessional, site specialised team working have finally changed the view that advanced colorectal cancer is an untreatable disease. Although cytotoxic chemotherapy is not suitable for all patients, widespread use in appropriate situations can improve survival and quality of life

Clinical presentation

Local recurrence of a tumour is more common in rectal than colon primaries. It may be identified early in the asymptomatic phase by follow up monitoring or may present with similar symptoms to the primary lesion. Blood loss through the rectum, mucous discharge, altered bowel habit, and straining are common features of recurrent rectal cancer. Pain and urinary symptoms are features of localised pelvic recurrence. Recurrent intra-abdominal disease can present as small or large bowel obstruction, and recurrence at other sites may be indicated by focal features such as hepatic capsular pain, jaundice, dyspnoea, localised bone pain, or neurological symptoms. Systemic features of weight loss, anorexia, nausea, and asthenia are symptoms commonly associated with advanced colorectal cancer. The tumour is often palpable on rectal or abdominal examination, and malignant ascites may also be evident. Clinical presentation About 20% of colorectal cancer cases will present with advanced disease About 50% of patients treated with curative surgery will develop advanced disease. About 80% of relapses will occur within three years of primary surgery About 50% of patients with advanced disease will present with liver metastasis About 20% of patients with advanced disease have disease confined to the liver

Which patients should be referred for palliative chemotherapy*? Patients in whom chemotherapy should be considered Able to carry out all normal activity without restriction Restricted in physically strenuous activity but able to walk about and carry out light work Able to walk about and capable of all self care but unable to carry out any work; out of bed or chair for more than 50% of waking hours *Based on the World Health Organisation's criteria for functional performance status Referral Despite clear evidence of the value of chemotherapy and the apparent willingness of cancer patients to have chemotherapy, in the United Kingdom only about 25% of patients with advanced disease are referred to an oncology tertiary centre for consideration of chemotherapy. Referral patterns and treatment policies for patients with advanced colorectal cancer vary widely in the United Kingdom. Currently many regions are in the throws of reorganising their cancer services as part of the implementation of the Calman report, A Policy Framework for Commissioning Cancer Services. It is envisaged that referrals to oncologists will increase considerably owing to the publication in 1997 of guidelines for managing colorectal cancer. Overview of management The management of patients with advanced colorectal cancer involves a combination of specialist active treatment, symptom control measures, and psychosocial support. Active treatment comprises an individual plan (often combining palliative surgery), cytotoxic chemotherapy, and radiation therapy. Current status of chemotherapy Many patients with advanced colorectal cancer die without having received chemotherapy. Chemotherapy improves survival by an average of about six months, compared with supportive care alone.Chemotherapy improves overall quality of life. Stabilisation of disease with chemotherapy improves both survival and disease related symptoms. Early chemotherapy treatment (rather than waiting until symptoms appear) prolongs survival. The outcome measures of the impact of active treatment have traditionally been survival, response, and toxicity. Alternative end points for example,quality of life, convenience, acceptability to patients, and patients' preferences assume greater importance in those with advanced disease, and they should now also be incorporated into the assessment of the relative worth of treatments. Surgery Palliative surgical procedures for advanced colorectal cancer are commonly used to overcome obstructing lesions and to alleviate pelvic symptoms.The liver is the most frequent site of metastasis, and in selected patients with no extrahepatic metastases surgical resection offers the only hope of cure. Five year survival rates of 25-35% have been reported with this highly specialised procedure (Cady and Stone, 1991). Abdominal computed tomogram showing a hepatic metastasis(arrow) before chemotherapy (top) and 17 weeks after chemotherapy (bottom); the later image shows a substantial reduction in the bulk of the hepatic tumour Radiotherapy. In advanced colon cancer, radiotherapy is rarely indicated. In locally advanced rectal disease, localised radiation may render some tumours resectable. Radiotherapy can also be effective in palliation of symptoms it can improve pain, stop haemorrhage,and lessen straining. In the absence of distant metastases, radiation may afford long term control of the tumour. Pain from isolated bone metastases can also be alleviated with short courses of radiation.

Conventional chemotherapy In patients with advanced colorectal cancer, chemotherapy is delivered with palliative rather than curative intent. For over four decades fluorouracil has been the mainstay of treatment for advanced colorectal cancer. Folinic acid is given intravenously before fluorouracil to enhance the fluorouracil's cytotoxicity. Large randomised trials of chemotherapy versus best supportive care have shown that fluorouracil based chemotherapy adds about 4-6 months to the remaining life of patients with advanced colorectal cancer. Chemotherapy delays the occurrence or progression of symptoms by about six months and improves symptoms, weight gain, and functional performance in about 40% of patients. Palliative chemotherapy in advanced colorectal cancer should not be restricted by chronological age but by fitness and activity level. Is failure to respond a failure of treatment? Less than a third of patients receive an objective tumour response complete or partial with fluorouracil based therapy. In a further 20-30% of patients, the disease is stablised during chemotherapy. The patients with stable disease ("no change" category) also derive a symptomatic and survival advantage from chemotherapy. Definitions for assessing response and progression after chemotherapy Complete response Disappearance of all known disease, determined by two observations not less than four weeks apart. Partial response Decrease of at least 50% of the sum of the products of the largest perpendicular diameters of all measurable lesions as determined by two observations not less than four weeks apart No changeLess than 50% decrease and less than 25% increase in the sum of the products of the largest perpendicular diameters of all measurable lesions; no new lesions should appear Progressive disease More than 25% increase in the size of at least one lesion or appearance of a new lesion

Which regimen?

Current evidence supports the use of infusional fluorouracil regimens over bolus schedules in terms of both toxicity and efficacy, but infusional chemotherapy is more complex to administer, requiring permanent vascular access technology or admission to hospital. In the United Kingdom a 48 hour regimen of fluorouracil plus folinic acid repeated every 14 days is commonly used. Ideally, chemotherapy for advanced colorectal cancer should be given within the umbrella of a clinical trial to help resolve outstanding questions of optimal type, duration, and scheduling of therapy.

Data from trials by the Nordic Gastrointestinal Tumour Therapy Group support the early use of chemotherapy, before the patient's condition deteriorates.

Tailoring treatment

The optimum duration of chemotherapy is unknown and is currently being tested in clinical trials. The current approaches are either to treat for a fixed period (usually six months) or to treat until progression occurs. Irrespective of which of these approaches is adopted, the overriding need is to monitor rigorously the effect of treatment in terms of response, palliative benefit, and toxicity. This ensures that any toxicity or disease progression is recognised as soon as possible and that the appropriate individualised treatment or cessation of chemotherapy can be implemented without delay. Chemotherapy toxicity Chemotherapy for advanced colorectal cancer should be prescribed by experienced oncologists familiar with the toxicity profile of the drug regimens used. Despite concerns over toxicity,currently used infusional regimens are remarkably well tolerated. Management of toxicities in the community requires close liaison with the hospital team, and severe toxicity requires immediate admission. The most common effects of toxicity from chemotherapies for advanced colorectal cancer are diarrhoea, mucositis, asthenia, and neutropenia. Nausea, alopecia, and anorexia can also be experienced. Diarrhoea can be substantially relieved with oral antimotility drugs. Mucositis should be managed with antiseptic mouthwash and prophylactic or early treatment of oral candidiasis. Neutropenia is less common with current infusional regimens but must always be suspected in patients with fever.Prolonged treatment with fluorouracil can produce painful blistering erythema of palms and soles of the feet (palmar plantar erythrodysaesthesia), which often improves with pyridoxine.

Patient receiving chemotherapy through central venous catheter in hospital outpatient department (top); and small, battery assisted pump, worn on the waist and used to deliver chemotherapy through a central venous catheter (bottom).

Cost effectiveness

In 1995 Glimelius et al showed that the overall cost of early intervention with chemotherapy in patients with advanced colorectal cancer is similar to that of no treatment or delayed chemotherapy, indicating that chemotherapy as part of the management of the advanced disease is indeed cost effective. Inevitably, it is becoming increasingly difficult for the health service to fund modern drugs to treat advanced colorectal cancer.The NHS is struggling to fund the new chemotherapy treatments that are proved to extend life by only a few months or to improve the quality of life only. Current controversies in advanced colorectal cancer. For how long should chemotherapy be given? Are new delivery routes for fluorouracil for example, orally and by intrahepatic arterial administration superior to conventional intravenous fluorouracil? Should newer agents with similar efficacy but more convenient intravenous regimens be used in place of fluorouracil? What is the optimum combination and sequence for fluorouracil based therapies and the new chemotherapy drugs? Is home chemotherapy viable? How are the new, more expensive drug therapies to be funded?

Ambulatory and domiciliary chemotherapy

The emergence of primary care health teams, together with developing technology, has allowed for more complex care to be carried out in the community or at home. Ambulatory infusional chemotherapy is administered via a small pump (battery assisted and disposable elastomeric infuser). The chemotherapy may be connected and disconnected at the hospital outpatient clinic by oncology nurses, or patients can be taught to do this themselves. A feasibility study of home chemotherapy has been undertaken in Birmingham for patients with advanced colorectal cancer. This shows that a nurse led service (backed up by oncology medical and nursing staff from both primary and secondary health care) is safe and that patients and carers find home therapy of immeasurable value. Early analysis shows that the cost of this home service is similar to and often cheaper than the current hospital based service.

New drugs

In recent years the availability of several new drugs has revived interest in the treatment
of advanced colorectal cancer. New treatments include alternative fluoropyrimidines, new thymidylate synthase inhibitors, new modulators of fluorouracil and also mechanistically new drugs.

New thymidylate synthase inhibitors Raltitrexed is a quinazoline analogue antifolate that gains entry to cells via the reduced folate carrier and is polyglutamated to a potent, long acting, specific inhibitor of thymidylate synthase. Its regimena short intravenous infusion every three weeks has similar efficacy to that of fluorouracil plus folinic acid and is clearly more convenient, although potentially more toxic. Liver with over 50% hepatic replacement by metastatic colorectal cancer Oral fluorouracil prodrugs and modulators Fluoropyrimidine analogues have been developed with reliable oral bioavailability. In addition, oral inhibitors of fluorouracil catabolism can facilitate oral dosing. Preliminary data show similar effectiveness and lower toxicity compared with fluorouracil.Given the convenience and potential cost savings, oral therapy may soon find a place in routine practice. Irinotecan and oxaliplatin Irinotecan is a camptothecin analogue that acts through the inhibition of a DNA unwinding enzyme, topoisomerase I, resulting in replication arrest with breaks in single strand DNA. It is useful in advanced colorectal cancer, even after resistance to fluorouracil has developed, and is associated with a survival benefit (about three months) compared with best supportive care. This drug can be associated with severe late onset diarrhoea, which must be treated immediately. Selection of patients, therefore, plays an important part in the safe use of this agent. The Colorectal Forum is a worldwide educational service for healthcare professionals working with patients with colorectal cancer. Its website provides news on conferences and events, recommendations on management of advanced colorectal cancer, articles and visual images, reviews of recent publications, and the opportunity to debate controversial clinical issues. It can be accessed at www.colorectal-forum.org

Oxaliplatin is a new platinum derivative analogue that crosslinks DNA and induces apoptotic cell death. It shows synergism with fluorouracil. The dominant toxic effect is cumulative neurotoxicity. Fluorouracil plus either irinotecan or oxaliplatin is superior to fluorouracil alone as a first line treatment for advanced colorectal cancer, with improvement in progression-free survival and, in the case of irinotecan, overall survival. Questions about the optimum sequence and combination of these agents remain and are the subject of ongoing clinical trials.

Intrahepatic arterial chemotherapy

For patients with unresectable hepatic metastases, intrahepatic arterial chemotherapy should be considered. This approach greatly increases drug delivery to the liver and doubles the rate at which tumours shrink, with tolerable toxicity. Owing to the complexity of placing the delivery catheter, intrahepatic arterial chemotherapy is usually administered at specialist centres. Current trials should offer definitive proof of whether intrahepatic arterial chemotherapy offers survival benefits compared with conventional intravenous therapy.

Further reading A policy framework for commissioning cancer services. London: Department of Health, 1994. (Consultative document.) Clinical Outcomes Group. Guidance on commissioning cancer services: improving outcomes in colorectal cancer. London: NHS Executive, 1997. Cady B, Stone M. The role of surgical resection of liver metastases in colorectal carcinoma. Semin Oncol 1991;18:399-406. Nordic Gastrointestinal Tumour Adjuvant Therapy Group. Expectancy or primary chemotherapy in patients with advanced, asymptomatic colorectal cancer: a randomised trial. J Clin Oncol 1992;10:904-11. Glimelius B, Hoffman K, Graf W, Haglund U, Nyren O, Pahlman L, et al. Cost-effectiveness of palliative chemotherapy in advanced gastrointestinal cancer. Ann Oncol 1995;6:267-74.

Supportive care

All patients with advanced colorectal cancer need continual evaluation of symptoms and appropriate measures for controlling symptoms. Dietary advice and nutritional supplements can stop weight loss, and corticosteroids may be used for their anabolic effect. Psychosocial aspects of care should incorporate evaluation of and provision for the needs of both the patient and the family. Supportive care needs to be tailored to the individual's circumstances and should involve the close collaboration of locally available palliative care services (both in the community and in hospitals).The initial contact between the patient and the palliative team should ideally be made at the time of diagnosis rather than at a crisis point when urgent input from palliative care services is required. Footnotes Daniel Rea is senior lecturer in medical oncology, Institute for Cancer Studies, University of Birmingham.The ABC of colorectal cancer is edited by D J Kerr, professor at the Institute for Cancer Studies, University of Birmingham; Annie Young, research fellow at the School of Health Sciences, University of Birmingham; and F D Richard Hobbs, professor in the department of primary care and general practice, University of Birmingham. The series will be published as a book by the end of 2000.

© BMJ 2000

Rapid Response responses to this article:
Read all Rapid Response responses
Palliating colorectal cancer with self-expanding metal stents.
Dr Steve Halligan, Consultant radiologist , St. Mark's Hospital
bmj.com, 23 Nov 2000 [Response] Colorectal cancer chronotherapy Joseph Watine, consultant, Doctor in pharmacy, Hôpital de Rodez,France bmj.com, 23 Nov 2000 [Response]

5th April 2001

Sarah Slater or Christina Osterling, senior registrar Dr Gallagher's team, medical oncology outpatients.

19th

GHF ward 9 am.

2nd May 2001

On day six after a course of chemotherapy, something switches on and Alistair can think again. As his mind clears so his body stops feeling exhausted and he feels better than he has for months. The terrible night sweats have stopped. Before the treatment he would wake with cold clammy sheets and snuggle up to try and get a bit of dry bed and eventually we would get up and change the bed or put down a towel and go back to sleep.

Awake at dawn to go to the toilet & hear the black birds singing in the quiet of the urban night and it is lovely.

9th

Barts 9 am.

After the Hickman line is put in (a minor procedure, but needing a full anaesthetic) a nurse sits and talks to Alistair as he is coming round, she tells him a story:

At The London Hospital (an old and un-renovated building with a reputation for vermin) *a patient is recovering from treatment, but remains reluctant to get out of bed. After a few days it is felt that she should be encouraged to do so, but this is met with some considerable resistance. A few days later she starts to display what could only be considered to be psychotic behaviour, the patient will not leave the bed 'because of the fox', psychiatric advice is sought, but still the patient insists that there is a fox under her bed.*

A few days later a fox is seen in the corridor...

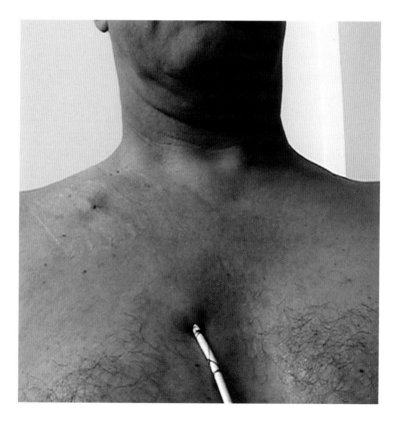

28

Sketch book no date (mostly Alistair writing)

Release form to look at notes. appointment with oncologist to discuss notes (Thurs. pm, Fri. any time)

Lung – when did they find the cancer here? how much is there? how long has it been there?

X-rays

LOVE

Fragments –

Family & friends, recent & past slow pans across/down so not all face can be seen/overlaps.

Medical info – details of imagery/text fragmented knowledge.

Emotional imagery – my reaction to.

1) Fragments (could include detail of my love)?

2) Available visual info.

3) Abstracts i.e. inside eye (space dots on surface) dream.

What you know – running along intercut in linear time as picture develops.

A structure for work & technology to fit i.e. book, vid, paint etc. with particular information & why relevant to that form.

Symptoms: sleeping, wooziness, lack of concentration.

Facts? trust – to run alongside as they emerge.

23rd May: Fax to Eric to check with friend at the Mayo Clinic

Dear Eric,

Alistair had the 'Hickman' line put in (thankfully, completely uneventfully), & after a bit of deliberation told OK to come home this evening. We went to the Fullers pub and had a pint before getting the 243 from the Clerkenwell Rd. Had the rest of your smoked fish in the fridge (yum), with a bit of salad and some good French bread from Gascon (and a wee drop to wash it all down).

Alistair is a bit woozy, but really OK and very happy to be home. Now watching the 'Cup Final' upstairs. I am not... roles have to be played and I am sticking to mine.

At the hospital, I have asked many times for the notes and had evasive replies. Finally discover a form signed by the patient is required before details are disclosed. (A. asked for this form yesterday but has not yet received one). So I took the blue nurses file left on the bedside and copied out the doses you asked for from that. I hope I have got them down right.

Weight height ratio.

CEA (carcinoembryonic antigen): specific indicator for cancer in the liver.

Response is usually measured in objectively (i.e. CT, X-ray etc.) reduction
in tumour size over time.

To be fair to the hospital, they have now said that we should both be present with a doctor to go through the file – a bit of interpretation of all the medical gobbledy-gook might be of assistance to us, I can quite see that they do not want people getting alarmed without help at hand. However, in this instance there is nothing left that is frightening that has not been thought of. But glad to be offered assistance... if/when it comes.

So here are the doses & stats (metric) Cycle No 3:

height : 180

weight : 82

BSA 2.01 (what is this ???)

day 1

Irinotecan	360 mg. (in 250 mls sodium chloride)	
folinic acid		350 mg. (in 5% dextrose)
5FU (iv)		800 mg.
5FU (infusion via pump)	2400 mg.	
day 2		
folinic acid		350 mg.(in 500 mls 5% dextrose)
5FU (iv)		800 mg.

Although I take a dim view of some of the patient/doctor protocols, it does seem that the treatment here is as it should be. But always good to double check. Thank you... really appreciated, let us know what you think.

Love from both. K

28th May

Had a consultation with 'the file' & senior registrar Dr Christina Osterling on Friday. Although did not give A. his file directly, she went through it bit by bit. CT scan images not present & she had not seen them, so could not comment on that. Record of 3 tumours in the lungs from April, no record of first blood tests (done at GP's request in April) but thought that markers would have been likely to have been high. Current blood marker CEA level at 845 after first cycle of chemo and at 442 after second. Said A. putting on weight was good sign. Next CT scan on 15 June & then a bit more detail. Although the general response rate to Irinotecan is only 40% and it is too early to tell, it does look hopeful.

40% of what? Of people responding, of tumour size, of life? It sounds reassuring so maybe that's why I have statistics without asking what they might actually mean.

How can dogs sniff out human cancers?

If Barbara Sommerville, a vet at the University of Cambridge is funded to test the idea, we will soon find out. Although Lassie never saved the day by excitedly leading doctors to a hidden melanoma, stories of cancer-spotting dogs abound. The first involves a border collie-dobermann cross that in 1989 evidently sniffed out a cancerous mole on a woman's leg. Then, in 1997, George (above), an explosives-sniffing schnauzer was trained to sniff out skin cancers. Despite George's reported success, dogs are not yet standard equipment in hospitals. "This idea still has to be scientifically verified," says Paul Waggoner, director of the canine and detection research institute at Auburn university in Alabama.

Sommerville wants to test if dogs can smell the difference between samples of urine from people with cancer and urine from healthy people. It's not a crazy idea, says Waggoner. Many cancers are known to shed specific proteins into the bloodstream that can also make it into urine. If they have a distinct scent and dogs' noses are sensitive enough to pick them up, it might just work.

Medicine has a long history of using smell to diagnose disease and groups at Imperial College, London and Cranfield University in Bedfordshire have worked on "electronic noses" to sniff out infections. Scientists tend to opt for sensors they have built because they are easier to calibrate reliably.

Waggoner says that it might make more sense to work out what cancer proteins can be found in the urine and develop a chemical test for those. An advantage of using dogs, he concedes, is that you don't need to know what the telltale protein or other cancer-related chemical they are sniffing is. This could be important if the protein or chemical was at such low levels that machines would not detect it.

Waggoner thinks the study should be funded if Sommerville has good reason to suspect that if successful, dogs would be realistic to use and lead to earlier detection. The study could also be useful in encouraging others to see if dogs can sniff out different diseases, he says. "Of course they might be barking up, no, I'll refrain from saying that."

Ian Sample

Guardian — Thursday 1st May 2003

The 'Hickman line' seems fine, A. is plus a bum bag of chemo rather than in a bed dripped up. Feels a lot different, better, but don't know what/how much response is psychological, being physically detached, autonomous etc. With this treatment we were able to walk up to Steve Hatt's and hang out in the garden looking at a wild Cuckoo Pint flower that had mysteriously emerged under the tree for Alistair's birthday.

I had a bit of a meltdown a few days ago, but OK now. We had a good birthday party, although Paul was tearful after the wine, so the boys had a big cuddle on the sofa. Both Hannah and Paul really lovely, around and about us, but also getting on with their things.

15th June 2001
Alistair – CT scan 12 Barts.
ENO *Lady Macbeth of Mtsensk* 4 tickets.

Sketch book no date – notes from conversation (Alistair writing)
1. K. loves A. / physically – tumours are a part of A.; K. can't change them, but it changes the perception of loving someone.
2. Satisfying love accepts rather than wants to change.
3. K. remembers standing at bus stop feeling delighted with her life. The feeling going – the future closing down.
4. Having to pull back into a short term future to make life exciting again. Projects. etc. look at feet, not horizon.
5. Not looking for trouble before it happens.
6. Making visual what you know you can't see.
7. Language very descriptive, but if can't be seen hard to describe.
8. Privilege of the objective/seen.
9. Symptoms can't always be seen.
10. Impressive, objective vs. vague, indeterminant.

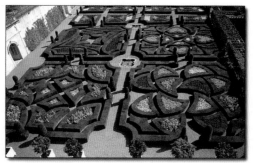

Villandry - les Jardins d'Amour

Septicemia smell: possibly from a change in the bacteria on the skin. Some bacteria cause a smell in wounds, but haven't heard of septicemia itself causing a smell.

Shivering with temperature: the thermoregulatory centre (thermostat) gets reset and muscular activity helps to generate heat. (Cytokines interfering - 'aiming' for the 'wrong' body temperature.).

Blue lips: drop in oxygen or constriction of small blood vessels.

Pethadine and other opioids are known to cause nausea/vomiting within the first days/weeks of treatment - it can be gradually prevented by prophylactic use of antiemetics. (This nausea is due to the central activity of opioids - in area postrema.)

Date unknown (sometime between March and August 2001)

Not passivity, but Alistair seems to know instinctively how to drift with the circumstances – many things that cannot be controlled, being able to live without control but not getting out of control. Spending the day waiting for routine procedures in a busy hospital and not getting impatient. Having to wait an extra 10 days for chemo because of low white cell count and getting on with something else. His ability to think on his feet, adjust, keeps things OK.

Friday 13th July

Collect flowers McQueens 10 am, get married Finsbury Town Hall 2.15, St Johns from 3, Sea View Hotel Whitstable.

21st August 2001

Got back from Cape Breton with Hannah, Alistair's postcard waiting for me from Villandry, we had stopped there our first summer together.

Alistair and Paul return from France. Within 24 hours it became obvious that A. was unwell. He had been very tired and was developing a temperature that rose steadily (and undramatically) overnight, he smelled a bit strange. I called Bart's and the nurse suggested bringing him in, they took some blood. The junior doctor thought he could go home at lunchtime but while we were waiting things took a turn for the worse. Alistair's temperature shot up to 40°C and he started to 'shiver' so violently the bed was rattling and his lips turned blue, finger nails likewise. The nurse gave him a shot of pethadine & he calmed for a while, then got very sick trying to find the toilet, disoriented, and lost it, vomiting in the entrance. I was following behind with a newspaper and caught some of it. Nurse Karen & I helped him to the toilet. A bad afternoon with shaking (more like convulsing) continuing for what seemed like hours & delirious. I think Christina (senior registrar) came by; he was put on a drip with saline, anti-sick and antibiotics, calmed and slept but still raging temp. Can't remember detail or timing, everything collapsed into a kind of timewarp of panic.

Septicemia is not uncommon with lines, develops rapidly (bacteria being 'mainlined' into the blood supply) always very severe because of mainlining and body's diminished capacity to respond.

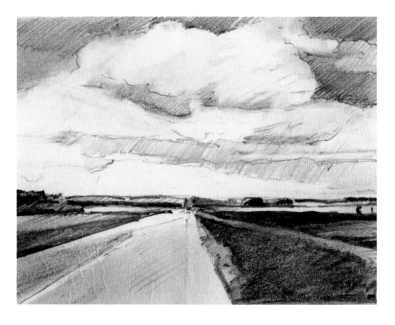

Sunday – temperature still very high, junior doctor somewhat posey said he didn't know what it could be, white cell count low so probably not bacterial... but the nurses appear to have a better handle on it.

Call Eric, they do not seem to be treating 'viral' infection, says to ask for anti-viral and specialist. Monday temperature coming down. Bacteria found in sample, a common skin sort, probably got in down the Hickman line. I feel very tired. Hannah's birthday dinner without Alistair, but it's easygoing as things seem to be going well. Tuesday, Alistair leaves hospital with antibiotics, OK but weak.

Tomas comes to build cupboard in our bedroom.

Friday a social worker calls from the hospice. This is a shock.
Good supportive team get Alistair to fill out disability allowance forms – should all add up to about £98 per week with mobility, or £60 if A. wants a car paid for. They also offer him free physio, aromatherapy etc. I feel horrified. This is like having death creeping up on us.

Later I get cross with Hannah for no good reason and cry a bit. When I talk to Alistair he is also upset.

23rd August
A. chemo no.8 GHF 8 am.

Sketch book no date – notes for diptychs (Alistair writing)
water
steam rain fog cloud
snow
ripples/waves
reflections/distortions
rain puddles pool stream river lake/ocean
rock – fissure cracks
large boulder churned over
rockface & mountain side

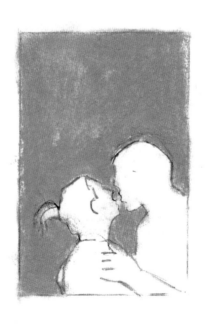

cloud/mist drizzle/fog snow
large broken rock
water running on the surface
rock in water
water turning and churning over & round
small rock smoothed
river running through

6th September 2001
Chemo 9

?
Something levelling (uncertainly reassuring) about the World Trade Centre. Destruction of concrete and steel – so efficiently taken out. Alistair has been discussing the structural implications with the architects at UEL (fascinating). The fragile self emerges as a constant, even in the face of illness.

18th
Alistair – St Joe's, 11.30 Denise, physio 12, reflexology 3.30.
(After this Alistair develops a resistance to visiting St Josephs hospice *'I want to live with the living, not live with the dying'* is how he put it..)

30th
Wasps v. Stade Français, Twickenham, 3 tickets. Hayley 6pm Matts Gallery closing party.

25th October 2001
F & V library. Call Claire & fix other appointments. Radiographer. Report from histology with ref number of tissue.

25th November 2001
Alistair – chemo 11.
Middlesex. Work on conference paper. 2pm Events Day meeting.

'Objective response' to chemotherapy does not preclude growth and spread of initial tumour or development of new secondaries.

16th November
Digital Aesthetic conference event. Post Alistair's private view cards.

18th
Stop the War 12 noon Hyde Park. Meet Anna at 73 bus stop.

November
Focusing on something painful can make it worse, or more intense – by drawing attention to it. When it gets overwhelming it feels as if there is nowhere else to exist – draw away from it and it recedes into the background – not denial, just pushing it away to get on with other things. The preciousness of the moment. Submerging in body pleasure and cerebral pleasure, to rescue us from grief.

23rd
Alistair scan 10 am Barts.
Open Studio show at Copperfield Road. P.V. 6-9 pm.
Really good turn-out, Alistair in his element talking to everyone, making everyone welcome.

29th
Collect tapes from Stanleys. Alistair, medical oncology clinic, Christina Osterling – BAD NEWS tumours growing again.
Waterloo 18.53 arr. 22.53. £95. Library, Pompidou Centre.

13th December 2001
Call ACE; Wellcome (rolling project but deadlines); Henryk.
South London Art Gallery, Station House Opera.

January 2002
Difficult period over Christmas. Alistair has been unwell ever since the consultation on 29th November with Christine.

Called the hospital just before Christmas, Alistair running high

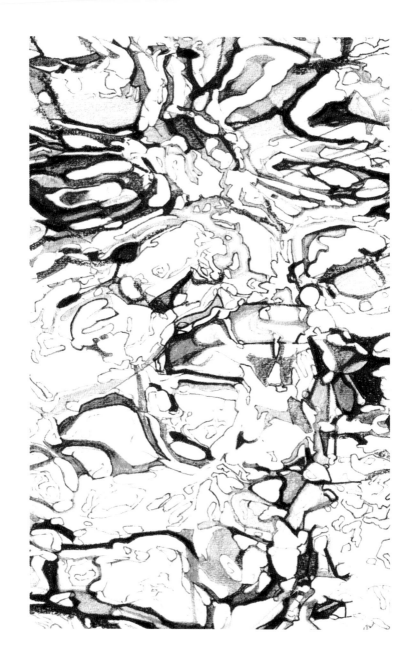

temperatures (up to 39) and feeling awful, doctor on the GHF ward said if he can walk please don't come in over Christmas. With the Hickman line in it could be sepsis (again). I am uneasy. Call the GP; Alistair feeling well enough to walk up the canal to her surgery, she gives Alistair a course of antibiotics and says call her any time, she will get him into hospital if he feels he wants that.

Slight respite for a jolly Christmas day. Andrea, Justin and (extended) family come over for a drink. Geri turns up early for lunch as he is avoiding Maureen who had arrived at Linda's; Hannah (having been to the boyfriend for 'breakfast') turns up with Guy and Carey and girls. Paul and Hannah organise after-lunch games, Ben cheats, us pissed, girls sing – Emilie's lovely voice – everything wraps up about 9 pm. Easy fun.

On Boxing day Dominique and Brian come over from Paris. On the 27th we take a long walk along the canal, up to the Angel, over the top, back down round Kings Cross and up to Camden, out at Regents Park. I walk holding Alistair, it is wonderful to be out again, I feel as if I am hogging him, his friends are here to see him but I don't want to let go, this is too much what I want.

Find somewhere open for curry at 4pm in Whitmore Street, the Frenchies seem tired, we go to the National (by tube this time) to see *The Good Hope* – very good. Alistair and I cry, but then we cry a lot now. The best day in ages, lovely people.

Alistair ill again. Have to cancel going to Stuttgart for New Year. Horst and Margret seem OK. I feel so bitterly disappointed I can hardly hang on to it. Must. Bloody tickets, can only get airport tax back.

Eric turns up with Debbie (D. not expected) don't feel like them being here. Alistair is exhausted.

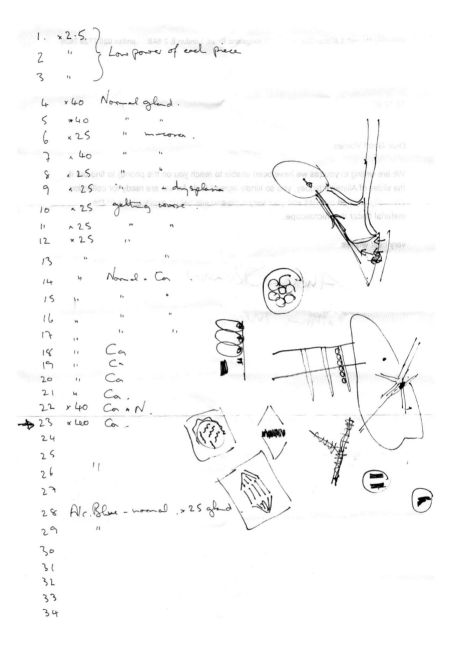

1. × 2.5 ⎫
2   "   ⎬ Low power of each piece
3   "   ⎭

4   × 40   Normal gland.
5   × 40   "   "
6   × 25   "   mucosa.
7   × 40   "   "
8   × 25   "   "
9   × 25   "   + dysplasia
10 × 25   getting worse.
11 × 25   "   "
12 × 25   "
13   "   "
14   "   Normal + Ca
15   "   "   "
16   "   "   "
17   "   "   "
18   "   Ca
19   "   C-
20   "   Ca
21   "   Ca.
22 × 40   Ca + N.
→ 23 × 40 Ca.
24
25
26   "
27
28   Alc. Blue - normal × 25 gland
29   "
30
31
32
33
34

3rd January

Geoff Vowles, histopathologist, interview with video camera 3 pm. Royal London.

No Man's Land NT 4 tickets.

Geoff was, or is, a rock musician. He has a messy office. Cartoons about the recent cloning of pigs with glowing fish genes and share prices of pharmaceutical companies are ironically pinned on the wall. There is no room for a tripod so I stand awkwardly holding the camera. He takes Alistair through a series of slides he has made for us from Alistair's biopsy. He explains the changes in cell structure and points to the different stages evident in the slides *'In tumours, the proportion of the nuclei to the rest of the cell tends to go haywire, nuclei becoming all different shapes and sizes and a lot more energy going into dividing and being out of control'.*

They are using an old slide-magnifying device, which shutters across loading one image at a time.

Geoff: *'...one of the problems is always that we are looking at something in two dimensions when it is three dimensional and dynamic...'*

Alistair: *'Can I ask you about the levels of magnification?'*

Geoff : *'It's difficult to say in a photograph, I've taken these with a x25 objective but the camera is adding on magnification...probably around x 80 when you put it into the projector.'*

Alistair: *'Architects use 1:100 ...'*

Alistair asks about the colour

Geoff: *'When we cut through a slice* (of biopsy material) *you can't see anything in it, it's just clear, we put dyes on it, generally two dyes: haemotoxylin which stains the nuclei...blue and then the rest of the cell contents stain up with eosin...in a mixture of pinks, but we've also got a whole load of stains that we can use to look at special components of tissue, for instance this is a stain I use for looking at mucin.'* (Alcian blue)

868 articles match
your search
"cancers".

Presenting articles
1 to 10
here.

Click on title to
view.

? January

We have been talking about imaging processes – genome sequencings are versions of bar codes, vertical ones look like Briget Riley paintings, and longer ones like Barnet Newman's etc. etc, except the medical imagery is very specifically indexical, perhaps borrowing from visual conventions of art/graphics, but leaving aside abstract ideas of absorption, as the response to the image itself is irrelevant, ho hum. The meeting with Geoff extends this conversation, with ideas of pigment and lenses, processes that seem mutually historical.

'Absorbtion' refers to a period when painting was considered in 'modernist' terms, and it remains useful as a way of describing a perception of painting as autonomous object. 'Indexical' is a conceptual approach where meaning is referred to outside of the object itself.

Alistair felt that art did not often get credited for marking out new territories. During the autumn of 2001 we had been to a series of science/art lectures organised by Rob La Frenais and Tracy Warr where one die-hard empiricist had claimed that art had no significance for science. Incensed Alistair said '*What about the Buckie gene?*' (after Buckminster Fullers's geodesic structure).
In the current hanging at Tate Modern physicist Richard Taylor comments '*Pollock's genius lay in his ability to paint such intricate fractle patterns so precisely and to do so twenty-five years before their scientific discovery.*' Alistair would have loved that.

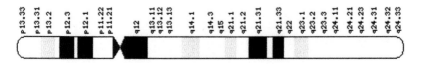

Platinum analogs knot up a cancer cell's DNA strands, which results in two different anti-cancer effects. First, knotting prevents the DNA from being properly copied. Cells that attempt to reproduce themselves but fail to copy their DNA will eventually die. Second, written along the DNA strands are the instructions to make molecules that a cell needs to survive. When the strands are knotted up, the instructions cannot be read, the molecules cannot be made, and the cell dies. Oxaliplatin is a platinum analog with demonstrated effectiveness in treating colorectal cancers. Oxaliplatin fights cancer when administered alone. 20- 25% of previously untreated patients respond to oxaliplatin. In addition, 10% of patients who have already failed to respond to 5-FU respond to oxaliplatin. Oxaliplatin also fights cancer in combination with other drugs. Several small studies have evaluated oxaliplatin combined with 5-FU/leucovorin. Each study involved >50 patients with colorectal cancers that had spread to other parts of their bodies. The patients had already undergone treatment with other anti-cancer drugs, making them less likely to respond to additional drug treatments, but they still enjoyed response rates of 20-58%. One study, involving 200 patients who had not previously been treated with drugs, tested oxaliplatin plus 5-FU/leucovorin versus 5-FU/leucovorin alone. 53% of patients responded to oxaliplatin plus 5-FU/leucovorin while only 12% responded to 5-FU/leucovorin without oxaliplatin. However, there was no difference in overall survival between these two groups. 5-10% of patients taking oxaliplatin experience vomiting but this can usually be treated with the proper medications. Reduced blood cell production occurs in about 5% of patients. The most common side effect of oxaliplatin, and the one that limits the amount of the drug that can be taken, is malfunctioning of the nervous system. This may be experienced as abnormal sensations and/or muscular weakness and occurs in up to 15% of patients. Rarely, unusual sensations in the throat can occur that are often triggered by exposure to cold food and beverages. These symptoms are easily remedied by avoiding the causative agents.
Drugs in this class: (View detailed list)
Drug Name Synonyms Oxaliplatin Eloxatin; Eloxatine

Friday 11th January

X-ray OK, Christine confirms chemo with Oxaliplatin starts next Friday. Go to Hammersmith Hospital to see Henryk and his PET scans/amino acid research, with video camera.

Henryk gives us some of the imaging processes he has been using in his work; 3D animated body rotations. As well as the tumour sites, the radio-active substance shows up the bladder as a black blodge.

Weekend – Alistair very tired, temperature fluctuating (up to 38 but not higher).

Alistair has managed to go to work, is absolutely exhausted, achy, soaking night sweats.

14th

Phone Royal Free re. clinical trials. Good and open talk with research doctor, but none appropriate.

Friday 18th

Alistair chemo no.1 Oxalyplatin & 5FU.

Alistair is very tearful in the hospital, must be fucking scared. We seem to take it in turns for complete meltdown.

I need to go at 10.30 to get to a meeting at Live Art Development Agency. On the way out of the ward I ask the nurse assigned to Alistair if she might see him, as he is rather upset and has been waiting a considerable time without starting any treatment (I feel cross but hope I haven't done it with too much mouth about me).

When I get back A. feeling better. The nurse sat with him in a side room and spent time in comforting and small talk to calm him down.

Alistair's funny story for the day:

> *'While waiting for chemo several patients announce boredom, one particular male draws attention to himself, so nurse comes over to chat, asks him how his treatment is going... and then*

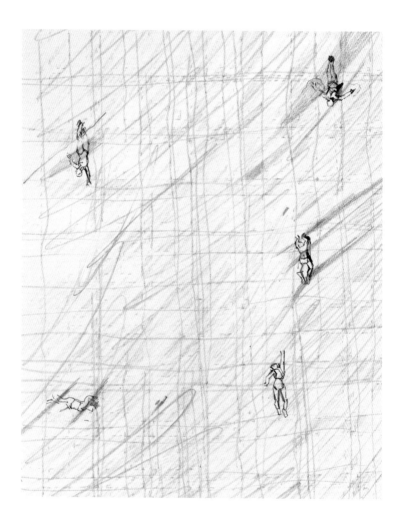

inquires whether he's ever thought of trying spiritual and/or faith healing. The patient looks quizzical and says he hadn't, so the nurse asks if he would like to meet another patient who found it helpful. She brings her over and introduces him with the words 'if I were in your shoes I would be clutching at s....' – she realises what she is saying and stops abruptly.'

When Alistair told it, it was funny and he insists I include it in this diary. I suppose when everyone is walking on eggshells, someone is bound to come out with the unmentionable. Out of context it is deeply unfunny, and writing it down does not seem to make it more amusing.

20th January
Willy Docherty, Matts Gallery 2-5.

31st
Barts. Alistair – Christina: clinical trials? 2nd opinion?
Masurca Fogo Pina Baush. 7.30 restricted view £38ea.

1st February 2002
Jeremy Steel on the day ward when A. in for chemo 2. Good talk with him, he says some interesting things in relation to interpreting symptoms, sweats and increase in markers could be the immune system kicking in, or could be bad news, big picture only possible after a number of weeks of relative factors. Strangely reassuring in spite of ambiguous interpretation. His openness feels honest and we hope, when Christina goes, to be able to see more of him. Treats Alistair as equal, not a dummy patient and likes to chat about art.

10th
Been mulling over visit to the clinic on Thursday pm. The bureaucracy at the hospital is appalling. V. chaotic. as usual two/three hour queues for the appointment, not knowing which doctor will see Alistair.

Cancer cure from Zulu

British researchers hail miracle medicine from tree bark extract used as a charm to ward off enemies in South Africa

by Robin McKie

Science Editor

BRITISH scientists last night revealed a dramatic success in the fight against cancer in which they used a radical new drug to starve tumours of oxygen.

The drug, combretastatin A4 – based on a tree bark extract used by Zulu warriors as a charm to ward off their enemies – cuts the supply of oxygen-laden blood to the cancers without causing serious side effects to patients, the researchers reported.

This is the most encouraging clinical result yet reported on drugs that try to block blood supplies rather than those that destroy cancerous tissue.

'I am very chuffed with this success,' said Professor Gordon McVie, director of the Cancer Research Campaign, which has funded the combretastatin trials. 'We still have more work to do, but this is very encouraging.'

Three years ago, the DNA pioneer and Nobel laureate James Watson hailed the development of angiogenetic drugs – those which attack tumour blood supplies – as 'a major breakthrough' in cancer treatments. His claim was based on the success of Judah Folkman, of Harvard University Medical School, who had cured mice of cancer using such medicines.

Scientists could not report similar success in treating people until last night when Professor Gordon Rustin of Mount Vernon Hospital, London, told the annual meeting of the American Society of Clinical Oncologists in San Francisco that his team used combretastatin to inhibit tumour blood flow in both men and women.

Rustin told The Observer: 'Some drugs have already been shown to prevent new blood vessels developing around cancers.

'However, we have shown something very different:

> 'We can contemplate destroying major tumours instead of just halting their spread'

that it is possible to destroy existing blood vessels.

'That means we can think of seeking out major bodily tumours such as those in the liver, lung, and breast, so we can destroy them, as opposed to merely halting their spread.'

Combretastatin was discovered by Dr Bob Pettit, of Arizona State University, during a survey of natural medicines exploited by native peoples. Pettit noted that several tribes in South Africa use the African bush willow, *Combretum caffrum*, to treat the sick, while the Zulus use it

to protect them against their enemies. Combretastatin was isolated from the bark of the tree.

The drug was taken up by the Swedish biotechnology company, OxiGene, which manufactured supplies for the UK trial. This involved a total of 34 patients suffering from major cancers of the lung, breast and liver.

'Tumour blood vessels and normal blood vessels have slightly different structures,' said Rustin. 'The crucial point about combretastatin is that it seems only to attack the former, which means its side effects are limited.'

To demonstrate this, the team used magnetic scanning devices to measure the blood flow through patients' tumours and through normal veins and arteries. Then combretastatin was administered and changes in the flow monitored.

The drug reduced significantly the flow through tumours but made little

difference to other vessels. In some cases, tumours were seen to shrink even after only limited application of combretastatin.

'There were some side effects but no serious ones,' said McVie. This contrasts with standard cancer treatments. Radiotherapy and chemotherapy can harm healthy tissue as much as a tumour, a problem that often impairs their effectiveness.

However, neither McVie nor Rustin thought combretastatin – or similar drugs being developed – would ever be sufficient on their own to treat cancer. 'Even if we find we can use these drugs to wipe out tumours, a few cancerous cells will always linger in the body, and could trigger a new tumour,' said Rustin.

'We will always have to combine it with other drugs that attack the cancer itself. It should be a very powerful combination, however.'

McVie agreed, adding:

'This type of drug should be ideal for mopping up after surgeons have cut out a tumour.'

Both scientists stressed that further clinical trials were needed to monitor treatment with combretastatin, which was unlikely to be ready for clinical use for another five years.

robin.mckie@observer.co.uk

www.crc.org.uk Cancer Research Campaign.
www.icr.ac.uk Institute of Cancer Research

As it happens they are short-staffed and a researcher has been co-opted from the Imperial Cancer lab, very bright oncologist, research on ovarian tumours. But not used to doing the clinic, communication v. difficult. Also says that January's CEA markers were over 900 (although we remember Christina saying this kind of figure in early December) new markers at 2,000+, not sure whether to feel alarmed or think the data has some missing bits, opt for latter answer as Alistair is definitely clinically improving, night sweats reduced and energy levels returning steadily.

We ask if the recent x-ray showed new tumours on the lungs, as there had been suspected lung disease mentioned on an earlier radiologists report. The doctor goes to look at the one computer terminal in the corridor (they don't have them in the room). He comes back saying the x-ray was cancelled – no data. We know that it was done. Alistair took it up to the ward and personally handed it to the reception desk for Christina, who obviously saw it, because she had to confirm that there was no infection that would prevent the next course of treatment.

The next CT scan that Christina had booked has also failed to get into the system, so we go with a new note and take it to the x-ray department to make sure it gets there. Technician says she will phone to confirm appointment date week of 11 March. We must try and get Jeremy to agree to have the scans present at the meeting following this. It may not happen but we need to keep trying. So far no meeting at Barts has been accompanied by the x-ray material even when requested, due to inability of the different departments to access the appropriate files. Reports, but as yet no hard data computerised, old systems creaking badly.

15th February
A. chemo 3. Thank you letter to Christina. Paul & friends.

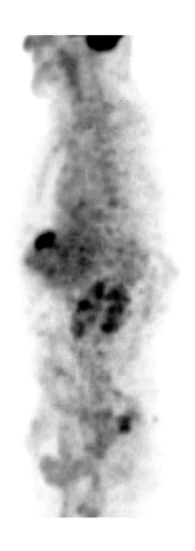

2nd March 2002
Weekend in France with brother Paul and Libby, ostensibly to buy wine, but really because Paul and Alistair want to be close. Walking on the beautiful wintry beach.

5th
Sina Dorudi interview midday – video recording OK. 7.30 Northgate, Ben.

Sina passes over a very eager researcher who has also been hoping to see him and gives us his lunch hour. He has a light office, his child's painting on the wall, he eats a banana.

Alistair and Sina really seem to enjoy the conversation, most of it centres upon public health issues, how Sina set up the colorectal diagnostic unit at The London, put in place specialist nurses, got funding etc, and why he chose his specialty. He is a curious mixture of pragmatist and visionary. Then they start to digress.

Alistair: *'It's the imaging gap between the high-tech medical imaging processes and the sense of illness. I still find that it doesn't relate to what it feels like, it's sort of space age, out there looking at the sky at night without actually understanding it. The debilitating things like the flu and not being very fit and running out of energy to zero very fast, Kate has to pick up the slack, and all the time I am trying to be, not superman, but I am trying to be who I was, I feel really sad and I can't quite get a handle on that and I wondered if you had any sense from your side of the fence so that I could actually understand it in some image way'.*
Sina: *'I am not sure I am going to be able to give you what you want, but I am prepared to see if we can arrive at something that bridges the gap between the stark image of a liver that's got metastases and a visceral response. I'd be really positive about exploring that with you'*

inside to outsid
Response

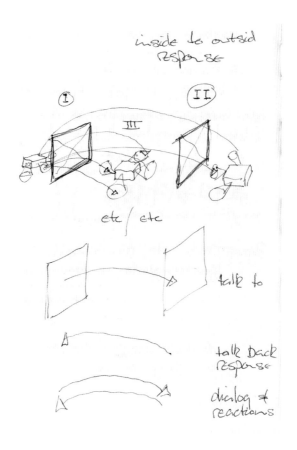

talk to

talk back
response

dialog ≠
reactions

Alistair: *'There was something that was said to me at the beginning, and I wish I could remember who said it to me, that to have a positive image about your illness and dealing with it would be very beneficial* (in coping with it) *and I took it away and I thought I'm going to visualise my illness & I'm going to try and visualise what chemicals do.'*

Then some general chat – where Alistair & Sina established our current knowledge of medical images seen and used to date, biopsy and scans etc.
Kate: *'...we went* (twice) *to see Geoff Vowles; the first time I looked and talked and you* (Alistair) *listened...*(you) *felt absolutely shocked and drained, and the second time we reversed that. You were in there, talking and looking* (I was observing this from behind the camera and this time it was I who)*...felt absolutely shattered by it... If you're involved in the process of looking at the image...it somehow becomes distanced, cutting out* (some of the emotional) *side of it.'* (by engaging with the material, not what it implies personally.)
Alistair talks about ideas of representing things from his position; perhaps inventing a persona to take the part of the cancer; using the various doctor's drawings. And plans to cast the Hickman line in bronze, as a heavy invasive object.
Kate: *'... it takes on this terrible weight in relation to the softness of the body'*
Alistair: *'not being able to cuddle and turn...'*
Sina (holding his chest in the position of a Hickman line): *'No one's ever told me that before, even women who have it on top of their breast...''*

We agree to meet again in a couple of months to take the imaging conversation further.

In fact we never find an occasion to do this. At the time there seemed a kind of irresolvability between the distancing of a medicalised or technological 'gaze' and a personal response, now they both seem fine as long as they are understood with their respective limits.

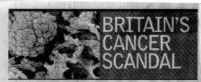

BRITAIN'S CANCER SCANDAL

In the second week of our campaign, **Anthony Browne** reports on why the latest treatments are often unavailable

THE DECISION will save money, but is expected to lead to the deaths of hundreds of NHS patients. But so routine have these decisions become in the new NHS that when it was announced last week it caused little stir except among medical professionals.

The National Institute of Clinical Excellence, the body set up by the Government to decide what drugs the NHS should prescribe, said it would severely restrict the use of the drug irinotecan for treating bowel cancer, which kills 16,000 people a year.

The new drug is now standard treatment across the Continent and the United States, and the effective ban means that thousands of NHS patients will have to make do with drugs 40 years old.

Professor Jim Cassidy of the Beatson Oncology Centre in Glasgow said: 'The decision by Nice to effectively deny patients the best treatments for advanced colorectal cancer is intensely frustrating. The only explanation is that it was primarily an economic decision.'

Dr Mark Saunders of the Christie Hospital, Manchester, said: 'It will be down to us, the healthcare professionals, to tell patients they can't have the best, even if they would benefit from this drug.'

Last week an *Observer* investigation revealed that, despite the Government's claims to have improved Britain's cancer services, patients were waiting longer than ever for diagnosis and treatment – this waiting so long that a curable cancer becomes incurable. Today we reveal that, even when patients do get treatment, it will probably be far less

advanced than that given to patients in the rest of Europe and America.

The Government boasts that the NHS is now paying for many drugs, such as Taxol, that were not available before. But the truth is the NHS lags years behind other health systems in offering the best drugs and radiotherapy equipment – often simply refusing outright to pay for them.

A typical example is Glivec, a 'wonder drug' that is the only known cure for myeloid leukaemia, producing remission in nine out of 10 patients. The Food and Drug Administration in the US registered it in record time last year, but it is not available in the UK. The NHS also refuses to pay for Herceptin, a drug that has proved effective for some breast cancer patients, and which has been available in the US for four years.

The denial of these drugs is leading to a two-tier cancer service: those with money are treated, while NHS patients are left to die. Saunders said: 'Nice was established to eliminate postcode prescribing. However, it will bring with it a new kind of rationing, "social class prescribing", where only those patients who can afford private treatment will have access to effective treatments.'

Anna Curaba, 60, from Roydon, Essex, has spent £60,000 going to Paris for treatment that even her NHS doctors say she must have. Seven years ago she developed breast cancer, which was treated in the NHS but which came back four years later. When she was treated again, the doctor gave her doxorubicin, a cheap 20-year

old drug – but scans showed that the cancer kept growing.

Her son, Joe, discovered that on the Continent someone with his mother's condition would be given the new drug Taxotere, which costs £2,000 to administer, 10 times the amount of the NHS drug. They visited an oncologist in France, who treated his mother with the drug. 'The NHS was going to let my mother die by making her wait three months and giving her 20-year-old drugs. But we spent £60,000 in France, and that cured it,' said Joe.

Often the drugs that the NHS is refusing to give to British patients are developed in Britain, with British money. For example, Cisplatin, a drug for cervical cancer developed in the UK, is available in the rest of the developed world but not here.

Professor Gordon McVie, director of Cancer Research UK, said: 'The frustration for us is that we do all these trials and prove these drugs work, and it's all paid for by the British public. But those who pay for it don't benefit.'

The Campaign for Effective and Rational Treatment, a drugs company funded pressure group, estimates that to give the latest treatments Britain needs to spend an extra £170m a year, giving benefit to 47,000 patients.

It is not just the latest drug treatments that the NHS is denying patients – the same is true for radiotherapy treatments. Britain's dated radiotherapy machines mean that many patients are denied 3D conformal radiation therapy, which targets the radiation far more effectively on the cancer. Dr Dan Ash, president of the Royal College of Radiologists, said: 'It's standard treatment in northern Europe, but a substantial minority of places in Britain won't offer it.'

Medical trials have shown that the best treatment for early prostate cancer is prostate brachitherapy – implanting radioactive material close to the cancerous cells. It is standard treatment in the US, but is only offered by a handful of places here. 'Lots of people who want it are being denied it,' said Ash.

The Government is desperately spending more money on cancer treatments, buying new machines and administering some of the new drugs. But doctors warn that, when it comes to the latest treatments, the NHS will fall further behind. 'The pace of research is speeding up – it's developing things much faster than the NHS can deliver,' said McVie. 'The NHS is struggling to deliver standard treatments – it won't be able to deliver novel ones.'

anthony.browne@observer.co.uk

www.nice.org.uk/article.asp?d= 28772

18th March 2002

The NICE (National Institute for Clinical Excellence) *'guidance for the use of Irinotecan, Oxalyplatin and Raltitrexed for the treatment of advanced colorectal cancer'* is published – it would appear that Alistair does not fit the correct criteria for their use, this makes us panic, Alistair is in the middle of his second course (Oxalyplatin) but thankfully there is never any question at Barts: teaching and research centres appear less restricted.

22nd

See Jeremy Steel late morning Paget Ward (see Barbara to get scans up), recording OK.

Jeremy takes us through Alistair's recent scans in the small side room off the chemo day-ward, liver still looks like a spotty dog, positions a bit changed from previous scans, some tumours shrunk from chemo and others now grown. Jeremy's special interest is asbestos-related cancers and he has some sharp 'health and safety' things to say about multinational companies use of workers in Africa.

We look at a strange 'key' image, in the bottom right corner of a big sheet of cross sections, which makes up a frontal picture of the body. Jeremy: *'That's what's called a scout film and it shows where the sections are, that's not actually an x-ray that's ever been taken of you, it's derived from the computer, the computer constructs that image from these images.'*
Alistair: *'Gosh, so they've flipped the scans sideways.'*
Jeremy (pointing at another scan): *'We are looking up at your upper body stump, if you were chopped in half.'*

28th

Alistair – chemo no. 6.
Deadline for Curtis, Hildamarie goes, ~~Hannah skiing.~~

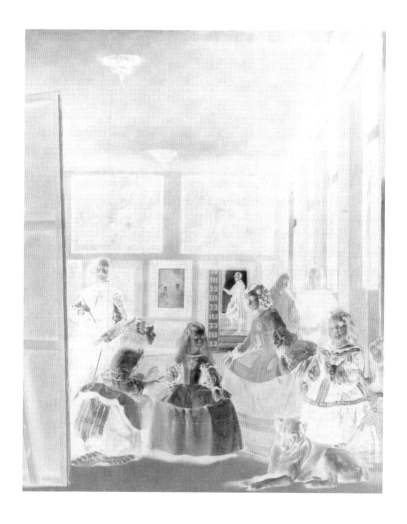

Spain 2nd – 8th April 2002:

Alistair has wanted to go to the Prado for years. This is also like the start of resolving unfinished business. We talk a lot about the project and shoot landscape. Water, rocks, skies and road movies.

In Madrid going to the Prado just for Velasquez' *Las Meninas*. The next day we go to see Picasso's *Guernica* again – it was returned to Spain after Franco died. Badly hung & not enough viewing space. Also see a Clemente/Warhol/Basquait collaboration show. Eat a lot of tasty things, drink a lot. Find an ancient sherry bar down a backstreet and then roll back to the hotel. Stewed dish of artichokes and beans etc. We eat so much Serrano ham Alistair doesn't want it again. And then to Cordova just for the Mesquita.

In the Alpajurras we have views from our hotel window to the sea with Africa beyond.

Lying together under the almond trees.

Visiting Julian, hanging out on the street with him for the *Burial of the Sardine* (a truly unrepressed spring festival in Murcia, with lots of naked dancing girls, etc).

We do things sparsely and with particularity, we are not really aware of this at the time, but it is as if we don't have time for things in general.

Plan some work around *Las Meninas*, very interested in different time frames and areas as if in/out of focus. When we get back we will start to paint on same canvas.

12th

CEA markers have gone whizzing up – blood tested 2 weeks ago at 1,580.

Jeremy said to stop the Oxalyplatin & look for clinical trials, gave us names at Marsden, Hammersmith & Royal Free to try, we meet him again next week to discuss what.

? Taste from platinum analogue chemotherapy.
Preference for bland rather than spicy foods: probably delayed gastric
(stomach) emptying secondary to enlargement of the liver with
metastases pressing on the stomach leading to reflux esophagitis.

Emotional lability: part of the psychological response.
? Possibly related to impaired immune response.
? Side effect of centrally acting medication.

Sod that.

Found a Nonesuch *John Donne* in Exmouth Market for £75, went to Moro for lunch, delicious, came home & went to bed, then A. snoozes, but I am restless, so I vacuumed house. Hannah v. concerned, (& she's feeling crap with sinusitis). We brought back a cake from Gascon that H. & Tom enjoy. All of us being calm if a bit shaken.

Thank goodness we had already had our lovely week in Spain.

Sketch book no date – notes from conversation (Alistair's writing)
Loss of strength (tiredness) legs and knees – falling over (once with child in arms) running on empty.

Tired, tension headache.

Sense of taste (chemotherapy induced) – a taste of metal on pallet – desire for bland food over spicy. Alcohol not very satisfactory (much reduced sadly).

Tiredness – sense of frailty (walking & esp. downstairs).

Confidence in motor mobility crocked. Recovery time very much longer (days not hours)

Easily emotionally aroused (cry almost at whim when thinking & talking about past & future).

Sense of my body – constantly check my liver (imagine pain when there is none & try to 'cover' when there is –'dumb').

Chemical – pattern:
A couple of days before chemo I am very stressy (taken a long time to recognise the fact!). Full course of chemo + 9 further treatments.

Increase in bowel movements. A number of possible causes: a panenterocolitis (inflammation of the bowel) caused by chemotherapy (especially 5 FU) also, decreased bile production secondary to bowel metastases leading to poor fat absorption. Metastases would lead to change in peptides produced by liver which affect bowel function. Necrosis of liver metastases could also release toxins which might increase bowel peristalsis (contractions).

Side effects of chemotherapy: malfunctioning of the nervous system, may be experienced as abnormal sensations and/or muscular weakness.

Liver enlargement: might be due to acute inflammatory response to chemotherapy, as effect or side effect.

Days 1, 2 & 3 – night sweats that leave a 'scene of the crime' silhouette on the bed in sweat.

Hickman line makes me feel vulnerable.

I find this hard – just recalling the symptoms, it's not where I try to place my mind day 3 + – continued metallic taste – affects both food & drink.

Toilet habits – more often & when you got to go you got to GO! (at any time of day or night).

On day 3 feeling of getting better – tingle in finger ends, lips & nose gets slightly less.

I have to avoid anyone with any minor sickness as my immune system is down till day 7/8 (I picked up a bug once – nurse said this is normal during chemo – & I was in hospital 3 days dripped up and out of it with fever Kate thought I was about to die.)

Day 7 end of course – I feel fine but constant monitoring of pain – I want to live with the living!

(I don't manage to do enough work as I want & this can really wind me up).

I am finding that my liver tends to 'get bigger' at the end of each round. This worries me, but not the doctor when I mentioned it last. (I may not have made myself clear because I find it hard to focus/concentrate e.g. in the middle of treatment 9 that although the markers were up & down something else was down 50% MUST ASK WHAT NEXT TIME.)

This constant attention to bodily detail drives me nuts.

didn't know that she had died. I know little about her myself, but it almost seems to me that she came from the sea."

Varda thus immediately foregrounds her presence as enunciative source while simultaneously relinquishing all authoritative certainty. She marks herself as distributor of the visions we are about to see, but yet retains no power over those visions—she simply offers them to us for our own active judgment. This is a process that renders enunciation dialectical, calls into question the text's controlling force. Intrigued by Mona herself, Varda sets into play a number of contradictory impressions, visions of characters that she creates but does not control, and thereby reflexively comments on all fiction-

May be an actual fluctuation or be within a range where the values are essentially the same.
Possibly due to ? psychoneuroimmunology (emotions can help to create chemical changes) the one lower count in this sequence was after the trip to Spain.

25th April

Agnes Varda talk 6.30 Tate Modern.

We decide that *The Gleaners & I*, is our favourite documentary, we saw it for the third time last week. Aspects of it have become a kind of model for this work. Both very excited to listen to her in person.

> *The Gleaners & I*, looks at people living on the margins, by choice or by misfortune. Gleaners in cities and of the fields, using the left-overs, the meanness and kindness encountered. Varda openly positions herself within this as a gleaner of images and friendships, using her camera as gathering device.

26th

Dawn – ICA bookshop will take three *Volumes (of vulnerability)* tins, meet Susan at 11 to arrange display case. Paul's 18th birthday dinner at The Real Greek.

3rd May 2002

A. chemo 8. *Hygiene* bash at Pam's.

4th / 5th / 6th (small note book, Kate writing)

Edit tapes for the *Hygiene* show, I work on the computer upstairs after discussion with Alistair, he has a cool eye. Fun putting Harvey's new soundtrack on, forwards on one tape, backwards on the other.

5th

Markers come down (CEA 1180 on 11th April), Alistair called back in for chemo, markers go up again.

It's now a waiting game, will they come down again? Or will they go on up and up? Jeremy very kindly said I could call him on his mobile on Tuesday to see if they are escalating and we need to try and change course.

Alistair is OK in himself, brilliantly not panicking, I go and walk mine off in secret.

I have high blood pressure, feel like my heart is breaking – physical sensation, not metaphoric.

Date	CA Markers
5/11/01	235
4/1/02	927.
1/2	2120.
14/2	1380.0
25/2	1640
15/3	980
27/3	1580
11/4	1180
19/4	1810
3/5	1480
16/5	2130

No protein going in therefore body catabolises existing protein (i.e. muscle).

11th May

Wooster Group, 3pm Riverside row L 26/27

17th

Alistair v. sick 24 hrs. *Hygiene* show Private View.

Our work is shown on two flat screens: crap speakers, so our carefully edited interviews with the scientists at the School of Hygiene and Tropical Medicine on issues of clean water get lost. Pictures look fine though, and no one worried about shit shot (unlike the reception we got at LUX).

Alistair arrives and turns back feeling terrible. Face the PV alone.

29th

I am awake tonight. Another scan later today. It has been hard to tell if the current exhaustion is down to the reaction to the Oxalyplatin or if the cancer is worse, certainly the CEA markers do not seem to be encouraging.

I mentioned that there were things I had written and thought that I had not let him know for fear of upsetting him. He said he had done the same, he says his liver is not right but does not say more. We both agree that we will be brave enough to share these things so I copy this from my private notebook, it was written a while back:

'Very, very gradual muscle wasting, (Alistair's) lovely footballer's thighs are gone.

It's an odd process, each stage I cannot imagine how I could stand any more sadness and then of course I do. I don't know if I want to slow things down or speed them up. Sometimes everything seems to pass infinitely slowly and then it feels as if it's slipped by without me paying enough attention.

I find I miss the past – the early days of our relationship seem so bright, the kids were so young and we so loved all of us and it feels as if it was such fun, so uncomplicated. I really think it was. And I miss it all.'

Police guard WHO official

John Vidal

A senior international civil servant has been attacked and threatened with death on three continents in the past three months in what appears to be a crude attempt to subvert his investigations into the pricing policies of the pharmaceutical industry.

German Velasquez, head of the drug action programme at the World Health Organisation in Geneva and a leading critic of the industry's policy of denying affordable drugs to poor countries, is being guarded by the police and told not to talk about what has happened.

Dr Velasquez, who is coordinating a WHO investigation into the industry's pricing of life-saving drugs in developing countries, was in Rio de Janeiro, Brazil, at the end of May for a meeting when he was attacked by two unidentified individuals and had his arm slashed by a knife.

Believing that this was little more than a mugging, he travelled to Miami for another WHO meeting on economic restructuring.

On the eve of the conference he was pursued down a road and attacked by two men. They waved a pistol, threatened him with death and kicked him to the ground.

As they left, one shouted: "We hope you learned the lesson of Rio. Stop criticising the pharmaceutical industry."

Dr Velasquez, a Sorbonne-trained Colombian economist, reported the incident to the Miami police, the UN in New York and the WHO's offices in Geneva before travelling back to Switzerland.

Ten days later he was telephoned in the middle of the night at his home in France. The caller asked, "Are you afraid?" and when Dr Velasquez asked him to identify himself, said only, "Lincoln Road, Miami".

The same man telephoned on the eve of a meeting of the World Commerce Organisation, where Dr Velasquez was due to talk about the right to health and the rights to intellectual property on pharmaceuticals. He was warned not to attend, and was again threatened.

His wife confirmed the incidents yesterday, and said that her husband had been told by the WHO to say nothing. The organisation refuses to deny or confirm that the incidents took place.

The WHO is split between those who do not want to embarrass the drug companies,

after assaults and threats

and want to work with them to reform their pricing policies in developing countries, and those who believe that exposure of their activities by campaigning groups such as Oxfam and Médecins sans Frontières is the best way to achieve change.

"It is terrifically sensitive," a source close to the WHO said yesterday. "There is an inflammatory situation in the global pharmaceutical industry. The trade rules are being rewritten and Velasquez is an overtly political civil servant."

Dr Velasquez has a long history of trying to reform the industry and has consistently

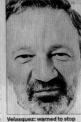

Velasquez: warned to stop criticising drugs companies

taken a stance in support of the developing world.

He has written many papers on drug financing in developing countries and criticised the power exercised by the drug companies. In the 1980s, with another author, he wrote a "red book" of drugs that developing countries needed, but this was unacceptable to the companies and was rewritten.

Oxfam confirmed yesterday that it had been briefed by the French police at Dr Velasquez's insistence.

"It is a strange affair," Phil Bloomer of Oxfam International said. "It is very crude. No one quite knows what any-

one is trying to gain out of this."

An associate of Dr Velasquez who asked not to be named said: "I cannot believe any of the large drug companies would do this. It is not to their advantage in any way."

The only known case of outright intimidation by a company was in the 80s when a whistle-blower exposed the alleged price-fixing of a Swiss company to the EU but was effectively shopped and later imprisoned for contravening the law on confidentiality. His wife committed suicide.

Yesterday the French police confirmed that they were investigating.

30th May

Hannah exam. Alistair CT scan – chest and liver 10.45. Temp over 39.
Alistair into Barts.
RCA painting show.

Black sketch book no date (Alistair writing for both)

> I remember that we were upstairs in my studio at the time, working
> together on a drawing/transcription. His lines are more assured than
> mine, although he is weak and he needs to sit on a chair

Las Meninas

How we read it/How Patron read it. Different interpretations through
time. How they accumulate.
Inside looking out mirror reflection outside looking in.
Time frame, focus, parallel narratives.
Painter, his world and his view concealed.

Parallel narratives
Man at door looking in (out of focus).
Painter – looking at the viewer (subject vanity).
Nun/scholar in conversation.
4 children, dwarf & dog.
Mirror reflection – showing viewers the patron.
Out of focus paintings on walls.
Inside the room & outside (suggested by light).

Pictorial Folds
Back of canvas/door opening in the bkgd.
Contained space/open space.
Geometry of the focal points.
Rhythms, patterns & textures.
Breaking space, holding up the space – perspectival games & geometry.

... ... undoubtedly reveals the ambiguity of a power that speaks of its own loss. It is that ambiguity, the value of uncertainty, that needs to be insisted upon. Then there is the man with a video camera, seeking to capture and visually enframe the world. The camera, the video, introduces the precise instance of visual power in which the reality and representation of truth are considered one in a metaphysics of realism. What fails to enter the field of vision, its classificatory procedures and representational logics, fails to become knowledge. The language of transparency and ocular hegemony coalesce in a subject–object relationship, and a unilateral understanding of meaning and truth, that reconfirms the subject; an understanding that moves in only one direction, from the I/eye towards the world perceived as external object. But the power of the gaze is also accompanied by an in-built failure, the failure to listen, to hear and to respond. It is a form of knowledge that tends neither to expect nor accept a reply. Critically to explore this path is to open up the process of anthropologising the West in order to 'show just how exotic its constitution of reality has been.'[24] This would be to excavate the theoretical disposition that has historically sought to capture and explain reality without itself being incorporated. Critical distance, scientific objectivity and aesthetic order is pursued while avoiding the paradox of the 'objectivity' of a specific point of view located in the partiality of a history and the partisan language of a culture.[25] The apparent freedom of the observer inadvertently reveals the intellectual enclosure in which she or he is unknowingly held.

Historically, it has been the look emanating from the centre that has guided a vision of things which has been unilateral and objectifying in its effects. But the gaze may be returned to render the observer uncomfortable. To register the possibility of such a return is to open up the disruptive distinction between the all-encompassing gaze – the subjective objectivity of the *cogito* – and a responsive vision that encounters resistance and opaqueness, disturbance and fuzziness, a murky reflection in the retina. This is to undo the critical distance between the all-seeing subject and an inert object – the distance that permits possession – with an interval that remains insurmountable, a separation installed and maintained by the finitude of mortality, by the limits of location and the position of a body, a voice, a history. In the passage from a confident

histories :
With
cannot sir
a telling
West: th
acquires
tions of
Western e
traffic betv
the occide
distance b
dread, alt
is not po
the hum
of comm
Henc
imity of
for all w
Western
more pre
this does
tual navels
also opens c
ment of we
power, incl
reordering r
categories
under-dev
the West
be rewrit
order to
tial criti
to how
wise, ar

20th June 2002

Saw Pain exhibition at Guy's Hospital, we both felt it didn't work as art, but recognised it might be therapeutic. Alistair felt it reduced spoken metaphor to literal objects – hot knives etc. and in representing these representations it just got further away from the point.

However the aspect of subjectivity in pain is pertinent, and there is a direct correlation in an attempt at imaging disease.

Friday 21st June

Coffee and fruit in bed to watch the 7.30 kick-off England vs Brazil.

Later.

Alistair said he had spent a lot of the recent two weeks in hospital trying to image his disease. He gets to the images on the inside of closed eyes – swimming blurry bits combining the back of the retina with the inside of the eyelids. He sees early Larry Poons paintings but with more detail, he sees a combination of structure and randomness. It is a bit like the magnified biopsy. When he tries to go in further he finds that he can't. Says his optimistic self that looks forward to things and gets the best out of what there is, just blocks getting in there. Fear comes in.

And also the sadness.

Alistair says he has not really been in pain, it is discomfort, but he often talks about the sadness that is lurking just below the surface, that as much as anything is part of his lack of image. It is as if he is looking for images that can have abstract emotional values. Obvious but complicated.

From my position I can imagine Alistair's tumours, but I am not sure if it is visual, it's more like texture. Little nodules. Geoff Vowles described the bowel polyp like an ordinary old mole on the skin; I imagine Alistair's liver with colon moles in it. The liver part like the stuff we eat,

Volunteer patients recruited to

James Meikle
Health correspondent

Cancer patients are being recruited for the first British run trials of man-made tumour busting viruses.

About 20 volunteers will be involved in the early stages of the experiments, testing the safety and short term efficacy of the treatments, which researchers hope might eventually be able to combat 95% of cancers.

They believe that injecting genetically modified viruses into the bloodstream will provide an alternative to radiotherapy and chemotherapy, which can lose potency as cancerous cells develop resistance.

The tests, by scientists working for the Hammersmith Hospitals NHS trust at Imperial College, London, involve mod-

test cancer-busting viruses

ifying viruses to work against tumours which have an inactivated version of genes that usually work against cancer.

Work is already advanced in the US on altering the adenovirus, a common cause of respiratory and eye infections, to fight cancers with an inactive P53 gene, including cancers in the head and neck, ovaries and bowel, and those trials have involved British patients.

However, the new research will involve using viruses to tackle a far wider range of cancers. They should kill the cancer cells but spare normal ones. "The idea is that if you make particular changes to one or two genes in native viruses you can make them less infective to normal cells but as infective or more infective to tumour cells," said Nick Lemoine, one of the researchers.

He and David Kirn, head of the viral and genetic therapy programme at the Hammersmith trust, outline the potential for the treatments in the latest Lancet Oncology medical journal.

Dr Kirn said: "Viruses have evolved over millions of years to express many of the qualities required for the ideal anti-cancer weapon.

"Viruses will target and infect very specific types of cell, multiply, cause cell death, and release more viral particles to go on and infect other target cells."

Rofecoxib (Vioxx) a substance used for pain relief which is also being studied for its ability to block the growth of new blood vessels to solid tumours. Nonsteroidal anti-inflammatory.

soft and smelling of blood. Slices before dipping in flour get merged with cross sections in negative of the CT scans.

I feel as if I can touch by remote. Put my hand up against his skin ever so lightly, feeling the difference in body temperature and something almost like a magnetic field between us. As I slowly pull my hand back I imagine the moles being drawn out by this action, disappearing, and the soft liver absorbing the gaps. I have no faith in this ability, but I can imagine it.

Perhaps the divergence is that Alistair is trying to represent what the image might be as a somatic sense of disease but this cannot be something externally observed. And for me, it is the representation of something physically external to me and therefore a viewing position could be imagined even if I am not sure what should be viewed. Maybe the visual aspect to both of our attempts is inappropriate (or impossible). Touch smell sound. A body map of someone you love is made from familiarity of the surface and a series of responses. Charting yourself is formed from inside to the surface and back again.

Black sketch book no date (mostly Alistair writing)
Trials at Barts? Dr?
What?
Trials at Marsden? Dr ?
What ?

Dr Slavin – said that after the infection has cleared, take a rest from chemo for a few weeks/months. Prescribe Vioxx, a drug that is good for arthritis and visit clinic every six wks to monitor the situation; will drop us a line.
Claire Barlow – appointment for clinic with Dr Gallagher and referral to Dr Cunningham at Marsden.

Capcitabine: an anti cancer drug that belongs to the family of antimetabolites. A drug used for over 40 years. (oral form of 5FU)

Bilirubin: synthesis by liver of e.g. crythocytes (old blood cells which are renewed every three months). A good perameter for evaluating liver function; too high = jaundice.

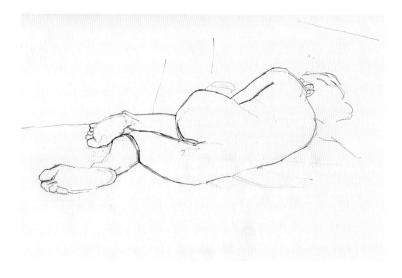

Dr Cunningham – trial at Barts is off. Not suitable.
Capcitabine may be suitable drug – chemo oral – with some side effects

What are/were the CEA blood markers on 30th May and is there a more recent CEA as well? (2,000)
Will you continue to monitor this at clinic? (yes)

CT scans

Why Cunningham not Judson at the Marsden?

Phone Dr Gallagher's sec. If don't receive a referral form the Marsden, note to remind Claire Barlow.

27th June
Marsden Hospital – Dr Judson for clinical trial? 10.30 out-patients, arrive 30 mins early for blood test, (CEA and Bilirubin). They think Alistair looks well enough to be eligible.
Notes on drugs trial CYC202 – cyclin dependent kinase inhibitor – prevents progression through cell cycle or XR11576 phase 1 trial, Topoisomerase inhibitor. (?same basis as Oxalyplatin & Irinotecan inhibiting DNA unwinding?)

Alistair says he looks up and sees me walking down the hospital corridor and catches his breath with pleasure, because I am his.

1st July 2002
Alistair is in chronic pain after we make love. I take him to hospital – he has septicaemia again.

I subsequently realise that this is the last time ever and it takes on disproportionate importance – I was slightly hung over, had a period, didn't make much effort, he turns me over, he is so beautiful. I remember this and wish in some way I had not been so bedraggled.

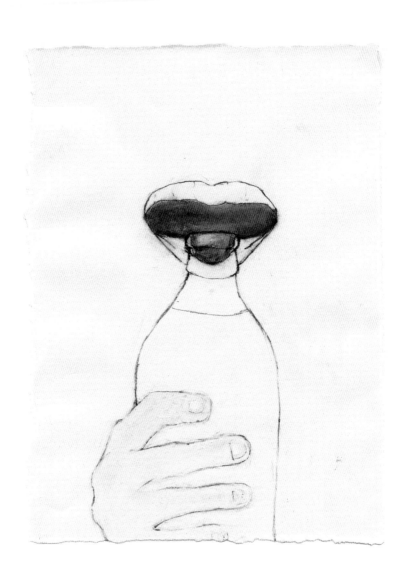

Black sketch book 6th July (Kate writing for both)
In Barts

Very weak 1st day of antibiotics after infection (from liver). Not eaten for most of the week, crying a lot. Pain killers.

Video questions:
Visualise illness as tumours.
Visualise illness as sadness/ emotion.

> We have been working on an idea with Gary Stevens about a cell production and mutation persona, as stand up comic.

How to represent Gary's idea of inappropriate objects (as in cells in the wrong place) such as table with outlandish place settings, watering cans etc.
Balloons – as organs – as cells.

22nd
New post short list Q.P. presentations
9.45 Rebecca Bowen (Dr Slevin) medical outpatients BARTS. Hannah to sort out broken washing machine. Ben 6.30. Capcitabine starts.

26th
Relearning your body as it changes – thin, so thin, with a great swollen ascites belly and flattened pink umbellicum. Sweet man, sweet heart. You have shrunk so fast your soft skin hangs in memory of your once muscular self, echoing those lost shapes.

And when you stand you are like a not yet fledged bird, all bone and middle. It is poignant, but not terrifying – that I could not have predicted. We choose comfort and composure. And you insist that you will say you love me with a smile and not tears. But you don't always manage it, any more than I do.

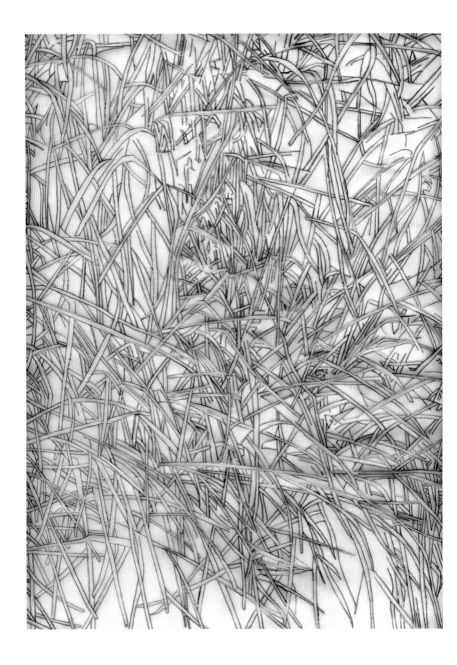

I wash your poor body, and something is beginning to push out from your anus but I don't want to say anything alarming and the smell of rose geranium soap soothes both of us.

29th July
Cancelled ~~9.15 clinic at Barts~~ spoke to Rebecca Bowen.

Loose leaf in sketch book no date Alistair's writing
(After Harvey visits, Alistair tries out a list of ideas for possible libretto)

First taste of fresh peach, the smell of cut grass, the call of black birds, lying still in the sun.

Friends, people, family. Treats, parties. Travel, histories, landscapes, cities. Sound, colour. Smell, taste. Sex, passion, lust, love. Games, play mistakes and daft events.

Friends, people, family. Treats, parties. Travel, histories, landscapes, cities. Sound, colour. Smell, taste. Sex, passion, lust, love. Games, play mistakes and daft events.

Black sketch book no date (Kate writes two words, Alistair the last one)

LIST OF EVERYTHING

the economic signature that was always hers, the logic of a testimonial idiom: her affirmation, her protestation in the name of life. She ends up affirming the triumph of life, as Shelley would have said, not the triumph of death but the triumph over death—not through a denegation regarding an anxiety over death (Sarah knew what that could be), not through the relinquishing of a knowledge of death, but, on the contrary, through an active interpretation that renounces neither knowledge nor the knowledge of knowledge, that is to say, the knowledge of the role that occultation or repression might still play in certain forms of knowledge. Whence the deployment of so many types of knowledge, the rigorous analysis of an intersemiotic and intertextual imbrication of speech, writing, and the silence of the body, of the sacred book and the book of science, book and painting, in more than one corpus, and first of all within Rembrandt's corpus, especially in the two *Anatomy Lessons* painted by Rembrandt some twenty years apart.

Twenty years apart, and there is always another anatomy lesson, yet one more lesson.

Here is the conclusion, where you will be able to admire along with me the precision of an analytical scalpel that does not forgo any knowledge but that also does not fail to reaffirm life—operating in fact so as to reaffirm life, but without resurrection or redemption, without any glorious body:

> The doctors of *The Anatomy Lesson* are gazing down at the book of science with the same attentive fervor as that found in other paintings (see, for example, Jordaens's *Four Evangelists,* mentioned by Claudel), where the evangelists are looking down at the sacred books from which they draw the confirmation of their message.
>
> In *The Anatomy Lesson,* the book of science takes the place of the Bible; for one truth another has been substituted, a truth that is no longer simply confined to books since it finds its experimental confirmation in the opening of a cadaver. The cadaver of Christ (for example, the one by Mantegna in the Brera Art Gallery in Milan, alluded to by the second *Anatomy Lesson,* that of Amsterdam) has been replaced by that of a man recently hanged, a purely passive object, manipulated, displaying no emotion, signaling no Resurrection, Redemption, or nobility. The cut into the flayed body thus also cuts into the religious illusion of a glorious body.
>
> The lesson of this *Anatomy Lesson* is thus not that of a *memento mori;* it is not that of a triumph of death but of a triumph over death; and this is due not to the life of an illusion, but to that of the speculative, whose function too is one of occultation.

Early July 2002 from video, taped in hospital bed

Conversation about how to represent disease:

Alistair: *'You know the sensation you get when you stare into the sun and close your eyes and you get things happening on your retina and you can identify patterns. I've mentioned to you before, it's the Larry Poons thing, the spaced out colours, in his early paintings, they were grid referenced so you had things pushing forward and pushing back over a systematic surface...'*

'Inserts of light blue against yellow background and oranges and greys and yellow that pan into this. I tried to think about when it hurts, could I actually get into that sort of space and I've found it really problematic, couldn't see anything other than an illustration till this current bout (of septicaemia) – and I associated it with balloons squeezed up together. Maybe the colour isn't important in that respect maybe it has to be monochrome. The (notion of a) balloon is good because it has to have a surface.'

Kate: *'Can it be acoustically represented?'*

Alistair: *'A wave. A lot of the time I've not been in excruciating pain because of the pain killers, but this constant discomfort which is weary, sounds of weariness, things running down, waves coming in, pulses and feeling flat, that has a sound too.'*

Kate: *'What does sadness sound like?'*

Alistair: *'It's not a sadness sound but it's like a trigger that sets off uncontrolled emotion.'*

Taped in hospital courtyard

Alistair: *'I do have this image of the pain which is like a trapped sequence of balloons. Sometimes I feel inside them as if I am physically part of those squeezed up things – that's when it's very painful, but its like all the time I am carrying this sense of these squeezed up areas which are on the edge of pain all the time. Balloons are quite a nice metaphor because they are celebratory party things, whereas these balloons are figments of torment.'*

Mechanism of action of slow release morphine: coating gets the morphine past the stomach acids and allows for slower absorption in the intestine.

Amitryptiline leading to semiconsciousness (eyes rolled back). These are extrapyramidal side-effects of amitryptiline overdose - direct effects on the brain.

30th July

Been a terrible few weeks with Alistair in and out of hospital and not knowing if he will be well enough for any further treatment. Now on Capcetabine and if he recovers some liver function they may try some Mitamycine (sp?).

On a low dose of slow release morphine but now trying to find a way to control the fierce and random leg pain. For ages no one had offered any explanation and it was very disconcerting and then Henryk and Astrid called by for a drink; and Astrid identified it as probably caused by tumours growing in the bowel and with all the nerve endings in that general region of the body, nerves can get trapped. After that I asked Anna (doctor from the hospice) who contacted the GP for some Amitryptaline and it was duly prescribed. Wrong dose left Alistair semi-conscious for several hours, eyes rolled back and mouth open, he looked like a renaissance painting of a saint. I took some video of him and wondered if that was something we could use, or if it seemed gratuitously mawkish. His skin colour was OK though, none of those grey tones or green underpainting.

Sunday and only emergency available and I couldn't bear to call another doctor who Alistair wouldn't know, and would quite possibly also not know what was going on anyway. Brother Paul away, Henryk and Astrid now away. So I phoned Eric to check doses. He called back & said it was far too high, but safe to let A. sleep it off.

Strange day, I washed down all the floors to keep occupied so I didn't panic. I decided that if he was in fact dying, at least he was comfortable in his own bed and getting him moved would have only been stressful. But it was tough. Next day I called Anna and she said he should be on about 10mgs at night (for neuropathic pain) not 75mgs twice a day, although that would have been the right dose if he was fit and using it for depression. (!?!)

Anemia: secondary to chemotherapy if leukocyte (white blood cell) count is very low. (? Could be septicemia could be causing symptoms.)

As the liver fails it can no longer keep producing the proteins required to maintain the normal oncotic pressure within the blood vessels. The oncotic pressure is what keeps the fluids in the blood vessels; as it falls the fluid starts to leak out and pool in the abdomen. Some fluid would also have been produced by the expanding metastases in the body.

Cancelled the visit to clinic because Alistair is still a bit drowsy this morning. Rebecca the new registrar at Barts said that was fine, just need to check he is not anaemic and they will deal with everything when he goes in for the 'tap' to drain excess fluid from his belly on Wed/Thurs.

Jeremy phoned to see how things are, we were both really pleased, as Alistair says, you have a friendly relationship with your doctor, but don't expect that to extend beyond a professional exchange. Jeremy said he would call in on Alistair on the ward Thursday, now he's a consultant he's at Newham on Wednesday.

Spiral note book (Kate writing for Alistair)
VET tape transfers.
Apple centre.
Stanleys – video stock.
Bookshop – Dan Graham, Larry Poons.
Bronze.

Jelly cherries in water.
Sponge, balloons.
Monochrome, salmon, dark to light.
Body shots.
Hand on body. Yours on mine, mine on yours.

31st
A. Barts GHF overnight drain belly

parietal

visceral

tumour
cells irritating
the layers & producing
inflame

fluid leakage

ad fatigue

fluid leakage

= bonds less
tight &
less permeable
= leakage =

outside

tight bond

(note taken into hospital)

for pain control:
Morphine sulphate
30mg slow release tabs   ONE to be taken TWICE a day (8am and 8pm)
Oramorph 10mg/5ml   as required, ONE 5ml spoonful
Amitriptyline   10 mg at night

chemotherapy:
Capecitabine 500 mg   FOUR taken TWICE a day
with Metoclopramide 10mg   if required ONE taken THREE times a day

other:
Lansoprazole sachets 30mgs   ONE dissolved in water in the morning
Dexamethasone 2mg   TWO taken ONCE a day
Bisacodol 5 mg   ONE taken TWICE a day
Docusate Sodium 100mg caps.   if required TWO taken THREE times a day
Nystatin oral suspension   if required drops FIVE times a day

It was important to take in a current drug list, because if they were not on the hospital notes they would not be given until the after the next ward round, which had been problematic in the past, this way I could be certain they were written up on admission.

Black note book (Kate writing for Alistair)

Talk about 'gate theory' of pain (WHO analgesic ladder) with junior doctor Steve who does the procedures, and then goes to the library and photocopies things for us.

Having tap: (to drain fluid) 'the prick' which is slightly sharp, made me want to hold your hand, as soon as I had reassurance it was localised, comprehended (hand held) dissipates pain (fall over, scratched surface, etc in this category). Felt anaesthetic spread and then it became warm. Track 4 on Miles Davis *Kind of Blue*

3rd August 2002

A+K *Picasso/Matisse* 10.45. Selina arrives am.
Selina brings Alistair a *Larry Poons* book that we haven't been able to get here. Alistair cheerfully decides to pay for Selina & Hannah's flights to *Documenta* since we now can't go ourselves. And Hildamarie gives them hotel money.

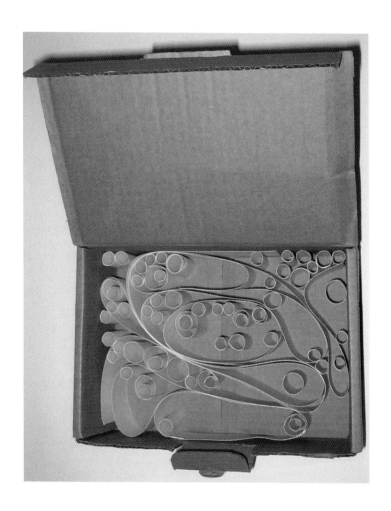

5th August
Dr Wilkinson 2/3 pm.

7th
~~10.30 Caroline Jenkins wheelchair assessment cancelled~~

8th
~~A.wellspring reflexology~~
Hayward – *Ansell Adams*; walk/push > London Bridge.

Hannah & Selina return from *Documenta* 22hrs LHR – with HUGE catalogue. Okwui Enzor as artistic director *Art as Global Culture* long talk with the girls about politics, art and documentary. They were unnerved by issues raised by Steve McQueen's film of mine workers, but enjoyed Isaac Julien's work. They questioned relative status of venues which they felt conditioned interpretations etc.

11th
Paul plays in Simon Rattle's Prom, Albert Hall 2 tickets, 8pm: *'Proud Dad.'*

12th
9am Rebecca, Barts.

16th
Big wheels fitted to chair am.
Coast of Utopia-Voyage 3 tickets (with Eric who has come to see Alistair).

23rd – 26th August with P & H
Had hoped to go to Greece. After holding it back for 18 months Alistair is clearly ill, but we go to Devon and Cornwall; to see the sea & eat fish... He is so tense he gets car sick on the way there, and we abandon our booking at Rick Stein.

Morphine patch: drugs that work on central nervous system have to be lipid (fats) based. Morphine is able to act on fatty tissue receptors, fat is soluble and therefore able to pass through the keratin of the skin.

Gradually accepting that we will take care of him, Alistair relaxes and the rest of the time is lovely. We both find it hard to recognise that Paul and Hannah are not only able to look after themselves, but are also very well able to look after us – sad to need it, but delicious to receive it. Alistair sleeps a lot and it is an incredible effort on his part, but we all want to do it. Burgh Island is fabulous, art-deco cocktail bar and the sea everywhere. Swim with P & H, it is very cold, I get 'deadfinger' – P and H find v. amusing.

Alistair is on Morphine, but relatively stable with the odd top-up of a liquid version.

Visit St Ives and look at art. Drive back with extra cushions. Alistair seems happy going home and talks the whole way.

Almodavar *Talk to Her* Rio

The young ones are out and we go to the early screening. We chat about
the witty way it raises thorny problems of carers and abuse, as I wheel
Alistair home.

29th August
Alistair– Barts for drain again.
Bronze casting.
Meet Mr Donaldson for 'discussion' with Hannah about school attendance etc.

30th
13.5 litres drained.
Alistair home.
Morphine patch.
Alistair hesitates as he leaves Barts. He has spoken to someone while I am out of the ward fetching Roger's car to take him home. When I return he asks me if I am really OK taking him back with me. I want him at home more than anything. And I don't quite realise the awfulness of what he has said, I suppose he must have known then.

Dizziness and low blood pressure: probably a drop in the tone of the sympathetic nervous system (which maintains the tension in the walls of the blood vessels) plus dehydration. This would lead to poor cerebral perfusion (blood flow to the brain).

CHRONIC LIVER DISEASE/ LIVER FAILURE

physical signs may be non-specific like fatigue,specific symptoms include:

right hypochondrial pain *due to liver distension (as liver capsular very tight)*

abdominal distension *due to ascitis*

ankle swelling *due to fluid retention (sodium and water retention as a result of peripheral arterial vasodilatation and consequent reduction in effective blood volume, the reduction of the effective blood volume activates various neurohumoral pressor systems such as the symphathetic nervous system and the rennin-angiotensin system resulting, thus promoting water and sodium retention)*

pruritus *with scratch marks due to cholestasis (could be obstructive or hepatocellular jaundice causing* **yellow skin, pale stool, dark urine** *as the serum bilirubin is conjugated)*

gynaecomastia *(breast swelling), testicular atrophy, loss of libido and amenorrhoea due to endocrine dysfunction (mainly altered oestrogen metabolism and treatment with spironolactone)*

confusion *and* **drowsiness** *due to neuropsychiatric complications (portosystemic encephalopathy: the blood bypasses the liver via collaterals and the toxic metabolite like ammonia, free fatty acids, mercaptans and excess of GABA activity alter the brain neurotransmitter balance that results in* **constructional apraxia, decreased mental function, asterixis** *(coarse flapping tremor) and* **foetor hepaticus** *(a sweet smell to the breath)*

skin alteration *like spider naevi (these are teleangiectases that consists of a central arteriole with radiating small vessels; they are found in the distribution of the superior vena cava- i.e. above the nipple line),* **palmar erythema** *(non-specific change indicative of a hyperdynamic circulation),* **clubbing** *occasionally and* **Dupuyren's contracture, xanthomas/xanthelasmas** *(cholesterol deposits),* **loss of body hair.**

1st September 2002
Alistair dizzy. Bad night.

2nd
Medical oncology 9.30. Alistair dizzy. Bad night.

3rd
Alistair dizzy.
10-12.30 programme meeting, Tom to stay with Alistair while I go in to work. Remove Morphine patch (as Astrid suggested) better night.

4th
Resume slow release Morphine tabs. Alistair dizzy but less so.

From video taped conversation early September
Kate: *'You were talking about the bubbles in the water bottle...'*
Alistair: *'Do we have a big flower jar?'* (He suggests putting cherries in jelly and melting them in the jar, to play with things to find images.) *'Ice cube size would be perfect.'*
We talk about how sound might represent things.
Alistair: *'Very much like the sound of moisture...'*
Kate: *'There is something curiously smooth about it.'*
Alistair: *'Body sound.'*
Kate: *'Yeah perhaps, internal sound, muffled, underwater sound.'*
Alistair: (enthusiastically): *'Yeah that's very pertinent, something submerged'* (he talks about Meredith Monk's music) *'She really captured the cold and winter and the sense of Northern Canada and the Arvo Part piece about passing time'* (or did he mean Andriessen?). *'They take you to a place which I imagine is true, that is wonderfully life-enhancing someone taking you to a specific experience, its magical – so I'd like that equivalence...'*
   Now I've got this off (dressing from the wound for the drain) *can I have a bath and listen?'*
Kate: *'Sure.'*

Confusion related to drugs and liver function: liver failure leads to build up of ammonia and other toxic metabolites of protein metabolism.. The liver is also increasingly unable to clear metabolites of morphine which are hallucinogenic.

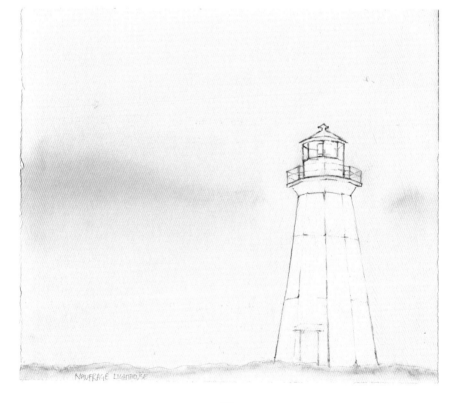

NAUFRAGÉ LIGHTHOUSE

Alistair also talks about the surreal images he has been seeing in things, finding faces in patches of colour, someone with a black hat and a baby goose-stepping, they sound slightly sinister to me but he doesn't seem to be worried by them. He is able to distinguish these (morphine visions?) from the process of searching for images for the work.

5th September
Amy (St. Joes) late morning, Trevor's *Dali* transferred from Edinburgh, 4 tickets (A, K, H, and Hugh) £36. 8pm. 1hr 10mins.

6th
Alistair getting confused. Collect commode. Annette am. Get tapes. Philip, Uschi, Anne Sophie to stay.

7th
Halve Morphine. Horst and Margret to lunch 1pm. Pippa later.

9th
~~Introduction level 1~~
~~Alistair Rebecca medical oncology~~ phone to cancel. Alistair too exhausted. Dr Emma (?) and Amy 1pm. Paul late. Andrea and Justin.

10th
Jack 11am. Amy after 2pm. Dr Wilkinson pm. Annette 4ish. Brother Paul and Etta evening.

13th
Libby.

Small sketch book 13th September 2002 (Kate writing for both)
My frail love, his mind is all a muddle, sight and body co-ordination gone wrong. This is so unbelievably hard.
IN DELIRIUM *'I don't know what it means to be zero, tell me what it is I should do?'*

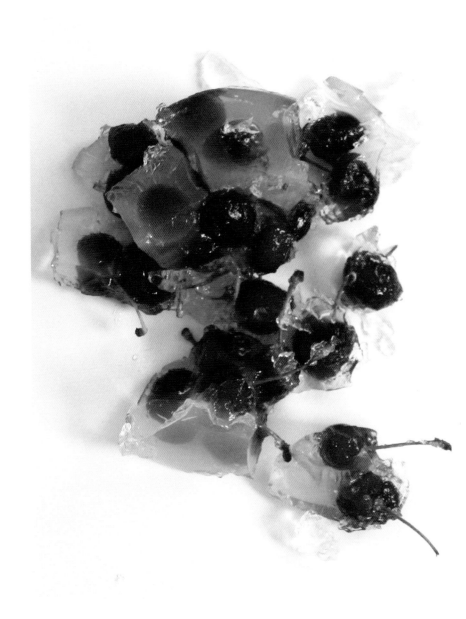

14th September
Alistair not able to swallow tablets, put Morphine patch back.

15th
Paul at 11. Brother Paul at 3?

16th
~~Teaching starts~~. Pain.

Unable to eat because of liver failure, plus pressure effects of liver metastases on the stomach reducing the effective size of the stomach. ? side effect of medication.

Unable to face meat: possibly because of toxic effects of protein breakdown products the liver is no longer able to detoxify.

Thrush: an opportunistic fungal infection following the destruction of normal bacterial flora by antibiotics or as a result of other factors. The antifungal (nystatin) breaks down the organism's cell wall.

September

A lot of friends and family come & visit, each time he says goodbye, he tells the person leaving that he loves them.

Paul and Hannah are around and sometimes come in to sit quietly near Alistair; I cannot bear for him to be alone now.

After a month the ascites has swollen up again, they drain it in litre sacks, clamping it off for a few hours between each, so the whole thing took a couple of days. This time just over thirteen litres, Alistair takes a joke sweepstake on this amount with some of the junior doctors.

Alistair gradually stops wanting to eat, for ages he has tried, mostly managing fairly bland things. Everything must be freshly made, won't eat hospital food. (Hoping to get some protein in; chicken broth, porridge made with milk, soft boiled eggs: can't face meat, and says lentil soup is for the winter. Nutritionist gives us 'tasteless' supplements, he doesn't like them.

As he stops eating he starts to get thrush in his mouth – try Nystatin drops & lozenges, they don't clear it and are disliked, so give up.

We go home. Alistair sleeps most of the time. Naked, close together. We have the TV and radio on a lot. One morning he is sitting at the end of the bed, he puts his arms round my waist as I am passing, leans his head on my chest and weeps because he loves me and is exhausted.

He no longer has the energy to be able to wash himself. He kneels in the bath while I wash him, because he is frightened that he won't be able to get out if he sits down properly.

He is unsteady on his feet, but still wants to go up and down the stairs by himself. Then one afternoon he falls, getting both knees stuck, trapped between the banisters. His legs are so thin they go in on the way down but he hasn't the strength to stand up again and

Odd mental connections: probably the result of a developing encephalopathy (brain dysfunction) secondary to narcotics or developing liver failure and circulating toxic breakdown products such as ammonia. Visual hallucinations: common side-effect of morphine.

Decreased ascites at end of life: ? secondary to decreased oral intake, also possibly secondary to necrosis of liver metastases.

Morphine smell on breath: metabolites of morphine not being cleared by liver.

Inability to swallow: as with eating: 1) pressure effect of swollen liver, 2) anticholinergic effect of drugs (dryness of mouth and digestive system, poor functioning of muscles).

Thread like capillaries: Spider Nevae-telangectasia (enlargement of the smallest vessels secondary to liver failure) also related to inability of failing liver to break down oestrogens.
Blue bruises and abdomen and upper arms: liver no longer able to produce proteins required for blood to clot, so small haemorrhages form.

his knee joints, bigger in a crouching position will not let him out. It is painful and frightening and after that he agrees to let me go with him. Willing now to be led like a child, he once forgets and calls me *'mum'*.

His mind starts to make odd connections, he sees images in unexpected places. I try halving the morphine, in case it is making this happen, after all he is so thin it must be relatively stronger than when it was first prescribed. This works well for a few days and then the confusion returns. I have been clutching at straws.

His belly grows again and then seems to start to reabsorb, in the last few days of his life ascites completely gone.

The room has a sweet dank smell of Morphine, which seems to hover around Alistair but is not actually quite on him; I can still smell him underneath.

Alistair can no longer swallow pills. Move to a Morphine patch, give up all other medication. Neuropathic pain returns, get the hospice to provide liquid Amiltryptiline (I have to bully them for it, but it is no good waiting till after the weekend and then going to the GP and waiting another day after that because the chemist will have to order it in).

Thread-like, red capillaries appear on Alistair's chest. Then some blue, bruised looking ones show on his stomach; and a few days later on his thighs. By the time he dies they are on his lower legs and upper arms as well.

He says he is feeling very poorly, his Manchester accent returns with that word, *'poorly'*.

Finds it too difficult to get onto the commode, is scared of me lifting him (although I can) does not like me to clutch him closely round the middle.

Skin hypersensitivity: ? related to jaundice, ? side effect of morphine not
being cleared by liver.
? Psychological: skin as a permeable barrier, often reveals (external)
symptoms related to (internal) state.

Acute sense of smell: smell is the oldest of the brain functions; as higher
centres function less well the input from the olfactory may be more
acutely perceived.

Pressure sores: loss of subcutaneous padding, breakdown of skin
weakened by inadequate nutrition.

Thirst: loss of fluid due to ascites leads to decreased volume in the blood
vessels, concentration of the remaining fluid stimulates the thirst centre.

Altered mental processes: 1) neurotoxins no longer removed by the liver;
2) drug metabolites no longer removed by the liver; 3) decrease in
circulating blood volume leading to inadequate oxygenation of the brain.

Thickish white mucus: secondary to dehydration and general weakness,
unable to breathe deeply and cough up normally (lying and immobile).

Skin is hypersensitive, thinks I have sharp nails, but it is just rough skin on my hands.

All summer his skin has been sensitive to heat, could only tolerate tepid baths (he used to like them really hot). His skin has become thin and delicate, as if so barely covering him, nerve endings all on edge at the surface. Smell also very acute, he likes the pillowcases changed several times a day so they are fresh.

Early one morning while he is in pain and I am giving him an extra spoon of Oramorph he tells me off for having bad breath. He is cross with me for various things during that day. Eventually I cry, Paul is in the room, I wish I hadn't. Later Alistair apologises, says he does not want to become like his father (angry with Alzheimers) I tell him I will try not to get upset, I do understand his frustration and he is much gentler with me after that.

He gets a pressure sore; we try sprays (they leave plastic gunk on the sheets that doesn't wash off) and then a condom-thin plaster.

He quietly says to Amy that *'This is hell.'*

Alistair becomes very wobbly, cannot sit up unaided, cannot coordinate his body. I need to hold the glass of water with him while he drinks. He is very thirsty. We work out a strategy of sitting up. He cannot move his legs easily; I slide them off the bed and each using our right hand to grab each other's arm, I place my left hand behind his back and lift him forward. We have to go back the same way because Alistair is uncertain where his pillow is. It could be either way. His mind is quite complicated, it is not just the drugs, everything has become re-routed. He is coughing up mucus, it is thickish and white. Hair is being left on his pillow.

The lump: shrinking due to dehydration and ? vasospasm (constriction of blood vessels); decreased peripheral blood flow secondary to cancer toxins and 'centralisation' of circulation.

Sputum yellowy brown: as mucostatis (mucus stuck in lungs) bronchi/alveoli are more susceptible to bacteria/fungi that will inevitably cause infection (e.g. pneumonia). The latter is 'visible' by coughing up discoloured phlegm.
A contributory cause could have been heart failure causing weak circulation, therefore lungs not functioning adequately.

He puts out one arm (he can hardly speak now) I wonder what he wants, and then he puts out his other arm and reaches me to him, to kiss me.

The lump that started to appear out of his anus is shrinking.

Last 48 hours
Pain. He can no longer hold his knee up, his leg hurts but he can no longer swallow the Amiltryptaline. I give him a shot of Morphine (according to Amy's instructions, that I have written on the back of an envelope) and call the hospice; they bring a syringe driver to deliver extra morphine continuously. Battery operated, it makes an annoying, intermittent noise even when it is under the pillow.

He cannot swallow anything easily, give him water from a syringe. The mucus he coughs up becomes yellowy brown. He repeatedly asks for a cup of tea, it is very urgent, he can't wait any longer and urinates a dark, dark fountain. I feel very sad and very stupid that I did not interpret him. Cup of tea = Want to pee. Somehow he manages to sit on one half of the bed while I change it and then roll him over onto the other. I still don't know where he found the strength to sit.

Last night
He can no longer swallow, not at all.
His mouth fills up and it is hard to breath through, I roll him on his side and I try swabbing it out, it doesn't really work. He is making noises as if he is trying to cry, I stroke his head and he is quiet for a while, this goes on for a couple of hours.
    I decide to give him an injection of Hyacin, one of the three drugs the hospice left (for pain, for agitation, for secretions) he seems

Breathing shallow and spaced out at end: likely developing acidosis as lungs and kidney no longer able to maintain normal acid-base balance in the blood.

Eyes would not stay closed, mouth clamped down: sounds like muscle spasm perhaps related to acidemia (increasing acidification of the blood).

Rigor mortis.

content to let me. It is 4am, although I did the morphine injection before, this time I want to absolutely know that I won't get things wrong, so I call brother Paul, he says put it in some muscle if I can find any. Upper arm still has a little, I tell Alistair it will take about half an hour, and I go on stroking his head, lying next to him, we rest a bit. Doze. At about six, again his breathing seems a bit different, he is staring up at the ceiling, drifting with his eyes open and looking quite content. I ask him if he can see something beautiful there, he refocuses so he is looking at the ceiling and makes a kind of quizzical expression, like 'What are you talking about!'

Then his breathing becomes more spaced out, shallower.

I sit and stroke his head until he stops.

The syringe driver makes a continuous noise, I take it out & take it downstairs without the battery in. The blood drains from his nose, it looks translucent. His head stays warm for several hours. His eyes won't stay closed, I am not bothered, it was just protocol to try.

Call the nurse, who calls the doctor. Libby phones. When she gets here, I ask Paul and Hannah to come home.

I go downstairs to talk to the kids, when I come back up his mouth has clamped shut on his lower lip. I am exhausted and lie down next to him to try to sleep, but I can't.

We all sit with him on and off during the day. Paul remarks that he 'is not there', he is right. When the undertakers come at about 6.30 I still don't want them to take his body away. His mouth is dry, his eyes are getting dusty. Strangely it is his gnarled feet with the footballer's broken toe that seem unchanged. My most beautiful sexy man.

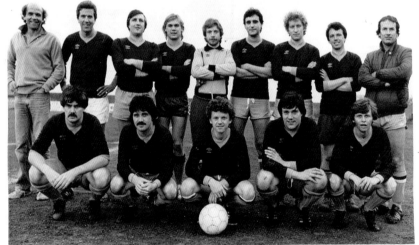

Roger Alton, Derek Scott, Howard Shaw, Robert Downton, Scott, Tim Jenkins, Phil Shaw, Sebastian Faulks, Tomas Shields, Ashton Chadwick

Nick Alford, Tim Evans, Charlie Robertson, Alistair Skinner, Ian Ridley

the body is created. A body analysed for humours contains humours; a body analysed for organs and tissues is constituted by organs and tissues; a body analysed for psychosocial functioning is a psychosocial object. But surely, the studies – analyses in themselves – which describe these historical processes can be said to be constructing a reality in the same way? .

Medical Commentary

mostly by Eric Clark and Astrid Schnabel.

Thanks also to Andrea Phillips.

Quotes and Illustration

front cover – Guardian Football Team and *Red Jelly*, Katharine Meynell
end papers Alistair's biopsy, Geoff Vowles
Birds, Alistair Skinner
Maharaj, Sarat, *Perfidious Fidelity - the untranslatability of the other*
Licorice allsorts, Alistair Skinner
Blue Bubbles for A., Katharine Meynell
Brault, Pascale-Anne & Nass, Michael, editors introduction to Jacques Derrida *The Work of Mourning*
CT scan showing Alistair's liver metastases
Colon & Liver drawn during consultation at The Royal London, Sina Dorudi
BMJ on line information
Alistair's chest with Hickman Line– still from video, Meynell & Skinner
How dogs can sniff out human cancer, The Guardian, 1st May 2001
postcard of *Les Jardins d'Amour*, Villandry
Road, Alistair Skinner
Kiss, Katharine Meynell
detail from *water/stones*, Alistair Skinner
abnormal cell division, Geoff Vowles
chromosome diagram (from unknown web source).
Kluke, Matthew, *oxalyplatin* from colon cancer online.
Swimmers, Alistair Skinner
Cancer cure from Zulu, The Observer, 13th May 2001
still from PET scan, source: Henryk Barthel
diagram for it's inside installation, Alistair Skinner
Britain's Cancer Scandal, The Observer
negative of *Las Meninas* ,Velasquez
Flitterman-Lewis, Sandy, *To Desire Differently, Feminism and French Cinema*.
list of CEA markers written out during consultation – Jeremy Steel
Police guard WHO official The Guardian 31.08.01
Chambers, Iain, *Culture After Humanism – history culture, subjectivity*
Volunteer patients recruited to test cancer busting viruses, The Guardian
Kate sleeping in Venice Hotel, Alistair Skinner
Tongue in syringe, Katharine Meynell
detail from *grass bank tracing*, Alistair Skinner
Derrida, Jacques, and Koffman, Sarah, *The Work of Mourning*.
diagram of how fluid leaks, Astrid Schnabel
'Cells' Kate's submission to box show, Alistair Skinnner
Naufrage (shipwreck) lighthouse, Katharine Meynell
Cherries in jelly, Katharine Meynell after an idea of Alistair's
Football team (source unknown)
Armstrong, David, *Knowledge of Bodies/Bodies of Knowledge, in Reassessing Foucault: Power Medicine and the Body*

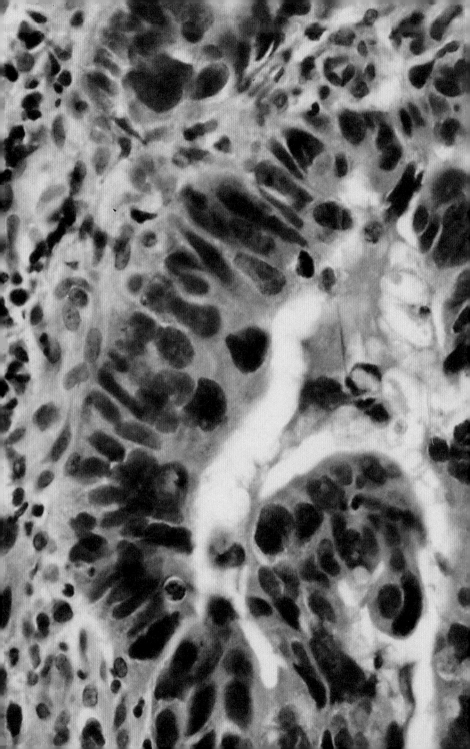